Intensive Diabetes Management

W9-BHX-510

American Diabetes Association. CLINICAL EDUCATION SERIES

Chief Scientific and Medical Officer
Richard Kahn, PhD

Publisher
Susan H. Lau

Editorial Director
Peter Banks

Director of Production
Carolyn R. Segree

Project Management
Christine B. Welch, Off-Press Publishing

Desktop Production
Margaret T. Webb, PhD, MasterWorks, Inc.

American Diabetes Association, Inc.
1660 Duke Street
Alexandria, VA 22314

First printing June 1995
Printed in the United States of America
ISBN 0-945448-51-1

Contents

A Word About This Guide vii

Contributors viii

Reviewers ix

Terminology of Intensive Diabetes Management 1

Rationale for and Physiological Basis of Intensive Diabetes
    Management 3

Highlights 4

Intensive Diabetes Management 5
Physiological Basis of Intensive Management Methods 7
   Normal Fuel Metabolism 7
   Regulation of Fuel Metabolism 8
   Implications for Therapy 9

The Team Approach 11

Highlights 12

The Concept of Team Management 13
Integrated Diabetes Management Team 14
Role Definition 16
Team Communication 17
Functional Considerations 18

Diabetes Self-Management Education 19

Highlights 20

Integration of the Team Approach 21
Diabetes Continuing Education 21
Assessment 21
Instruction 22
   Environment 22
   Planning 23
   Content 23
   Sequencing of Classes 23
   Approaches/Strategies 25
Motivation 25

Negotiation 25
Evaluation 25
Documentation 26

Psychosocial Issues..29

Highlights 30

Assessing Patient Suitability for Intensification 31
   Practicing Behavior 31
   Assessing Psychosocial Status 32
Assessing the Effect of Stress on Glycemic Control 33
Assessing Coping Skills 35
   Assessment of Diabetes-Related Coping 35
   Identifying Psychosocial Resources 35
Helping Patients Deal With Complications 36
Helping Patients With Long-Term Adherence 37
Supporting Patients' Behavior Change 38

Patient Selection and Goals of Therapy 41

Highlights 42

Patient Selection 43
   Patients With Type I Diabetes 44
   Patients With Type II Diabetes 45
Goals of Therapy 46
   Glycemic Goals 47
   Modifying Glycemic Goals 47
   Weighing the Benefits and Risks in Type II Diabetes 48

Multiple-Component Insulin Regimens 51

Highlights 52

Insulin Pharmacology 53
   Insulin Timing and Action 53
   Stability and Miscibility of Insulins 54
   Insulin Absorption 55
Insulin Regimens 56
   Multiple-Component Insulin Regimens: General Points 56
   Specific Flexible Multiple-Component Insulin Regimens 57
   Other Intensive (But Less Flexible) Insulin Programs 58
Insulin Dose and Distribution 60

Initial Insulin Doses 60
Insulin Dose Distribution 60
Insulin Algorithms 60
Preprandial Algorithms 61
Pattern-Adjustment Algorithms 61
Injection Devices 64

Insulin Infusion Pump Therapy 65

Highlights 66

Why Use CSII? 67
Initial Dosage Calculations for Insulin Pump Therapy 68
Insulin Adjustments 70
Diet 70
Exercise 70
Illness 70
Correction of Hyperglycemia 70
Risks of CSII 71
Skin Infection 71
Unexplained Hyperglycemia 71
Hypoglycemia 73
Wearing the Pump 73
Patient Education for CSII 74
Implantable Insulin Infusion Pumps 76

Monitoring..79

Highlights 80

Monitoring by the Patient 81
Blood Glucose 81
Urine Ketones 82
Record Keeping 83
Monitoring by the Health-Care Team 83
Glycated Hemoglobin 84
Hypoglycemia 86
Monitoring for Long-Term Complications 86

Nutrition Management...89
Highlights 90

Goals of Medical Nutrition Therapy 91
Target Nutrition Recommendations 92
Strategies for Type I Diabetes 93
Strategies for Type II Diabetes 95
Glucose Monitoring and the Nutritional Plan 96
Hypoglycemia 96
    Skipping or Delaying Planned Meals or Snacks 96
    Inappropriate Timing of Insulin Relative to Meals 98
    Imbalance Between Food and Meal-Related Insulin Dose 98
    Inadequate Food Supplements for Exercise 99
    Consuming Alcohol on an Empty Stomach 99
    Oral Treatment of Hypoglycemia 100
Facilitating Nutrition Self-Management 101
    Meal Planning Approaches for Intensified Management 101
    Carbohydrate Counting 101
Weight Gain Associated With Intensive Management 104

Adverse Effects 105
Highlights 106

Hypoglycemia 107
    Prevention 107
Weight Gain 108
    Prevention 108
Infusion Site Infections in Insulin Pump Use 109

Resources 110

Index 111

A Word About This Guide

*I*ntensive Diabetes Management joins the American Diabetes Association's Clinical Education Series, which also includes *Medical Management of Non-Insulin-Dependent (Type II) Diabetes*, *Medical Management of Insulin-Dependent (Type I) Diabetes*, *Medical Management of Pregnancy Complicated by Diabetes*, and *Therapy for Diabetes Mellitus and Related Disorders*. The Clinical Education Series provides health-care professionals with the comprehensive information needed to give the best possible medical care to patients with diabetes.

Intensive Diabetes Management focuses on the intensive management of patients with type I or type II diabetes. The idea for this book was conceived during discussions with colleagues regarding implementation of the results of the Diabetes Control and Complications Trial (DCCT). The goal was to present a practical guide for clinical care and patient education, with emphasis on the team approach to diabetes care and comprehensive self-management education. This book is a project of ADA's Council on Education.

All contributors are experts in their respective fields who are intimately involved in helping patients intensify their diabetes management. They offer the approaches to intensive diabetes management that they have found to be of most benefit to patients. They share their techniques for success, including altering treatment regimens and glycemic goals to the patient's needs and abilities. What has emerged is the most practical book available on how to begin and maintain intensive diabetes management. The contributors have based their recommendations on the results of the DCCT and the ADA's Clinical Practice Recommendations.

I hope that *Intensive Diabetes Management* will be a useful addition to your professional library and that it will inspire you to incorporate the knowledge and skills presented here within your clinical practice. All health professionals who care for people with diabetes will find guidance for implementing the improved diabetes care we know is so valuable.

RUTH FARKAS-HIRSCH, MS, RN, CDE
Editor-in-Chief

Contributors

Editor-in-Chief	RUTH FARKAS-HIRSCH, MS, RN, CDE University of Washington Medical Center Seattle, Washington

Contributing Editors	BETTY PAGE BRACKENRIDGE, MS, RD, Editors CDE Learning Prescriptions Phoenix, Arizona
	RODNEY A. LORENZ, MD Vanderbilt University Medical Center Nashville, Tennessee
	GAYLE M. LORENZI, BSN, RN, CDE University of California San Diego School of Medicine La Jolla, California
	BARBARA SCHREINER, RN, MN, CDE Texas Diabetes and Endocrine Center at Heimann Hospital Houston, Texas
	JAY S. SKYLER, MD University of Miami School of Medicine Miami, Florida
	SUZANNE M. STROWIG, MSN, RN, CDE University of Texas Southwestern Medical Center Dallas, Texas
	NEIL H. WHITE, MD, CDE Washington University School of Medicine St. Louis, Missouri
	FRED W. WHITEHOUSE, MD, FACP Henry Ford Hospital Detroit, Michigan
	DEBORAH YOUNG-HYMAN, PhD, CDE University of Maryland Medical School Baltimore, Maryland

Reviewers

MARION J. FRANZ, RD, MS, CDE
International Diabetes Center
Minneapolis, Minnesota

GEORGE GRUNBERGER, MD
Wayne State University
Detroit, Michigan

CINDY L. HANSON, PhD
Medical University of South Carolina
Charleston, North Carolina

DAVID B. KELLEY
Middleton Foundation, Inc.
Olympia, Washington

VIRGINIA PERGALLO-DITTKO, RN, MA, CDE
Diabetes Education Center, Winthrop-University Hospital
Mineola, New York

JULIO V. SANTIAGO, MD
St. Louis Children's Hospital
St. Louis, Missouri

DAVID S. SCHADE, MD
The University of New Mexico School of Medicine
Albuquerque, New Mexico

Terminology of Intensive Diabetes Management

- **Insulin-dependent (type I) diabetes mellitus:** A disorder that causes progressive destruction of the pancreatic ß-cells (insulitis), leading to a permanent insulin-dependent state. In most cases, type I diabetes mellitus is an autoimmune disorder.

- **Non-insulin-dependent (type II) diabetes:** A disorder manifested by peripheral insulin resistance and varying degrees of insulin deficiency. Some patients require insulin therapy.

- **Intensive diabetes management:** A mode of treatment for the person with diabetes that has the goal of achieving euglycemia or near-normal glycemia, using all available resources to accomplish this goal.

- **Improved glycemic control:** Lowered levels of glycated hemoglobin and mean blood glucose than during a previous course of diabetes therapy.

- **Near-normal glycemic control:** An average blood glucose level of 150 mg/dl, which corresponds to a glycated hemoglobin level 1% above the upper limit of normal for the laboratory.

- **Euglycemic control:** Blood glucose levels that fall within the nondiabetic range of 60–120 mg/dl, which corresponds to a normal glycated hemoglobin level for the laboratory.

- **Diabetes team:** A core of health-care professionals actively working with a patient with diabetes toward common goals of management. In addition to the patient, the team includes a physician, a nurse manager/educator/clinician, a dietitian, a mental health professional, and other specialists as needed, all experienced in the care of people with diabetes.

- **Basal insulin:** An intermediate-acting (NPH or lente) or long-acting (ultralente) insulin that offers slower absorption from a subcutaneous depot into the bloodstream, permitting a steady level of plasma insulin. This insulin dose mimics the postabsorptive secretion of insulin by pancreatic ß-cells. Also used to describe background insulin given continuously by insulin pump.

- **Bolus insulin:** Regular insulin or a fast-acting insulin analogue injected in relation to food intake to permit a rapid rise in plasma insulin level after a meal. This insulin injection mimics the postprandial secretion of insulin by pancreatic ß-cells and blunts the rise in blood glucose. Also used to describe the preprandial insulin dose delivered by insulin pump.

- **Insulin infusion pump:** A continuous subcutaneous insulin infusion (CSII) system that delivers regular insulin in an open-loop fashion into a subcutaneous site from a computer-driven, externally mounted syringe. Commonly referred to as an insulin pump.

- **Multiple doses of insulin (MDI):** A management strategy for insulin delivery that includes the use of three or more injections of insulin daily to provide both basal and bolus insulin requirements.

- **Lag time:** That period (in minutes) between the subcutaneous injection of regular insulin and its initially effective physiologic action. This period may be 10–60 min and is unpredictably variable from person to person and in the same person from time to time.

- **Open-loop insulin delivery:** A system of insulin delivery that is independent of the moment-to-moment changes in plasma glucose levels. This delivery system is the only type available to the patient with diabetes in 1995.

- **Closed-loop insulin delivery:** A system of insulin delivery wherein insulin is released into the bloodstream in response to the moment-to-moment change in the plasma glucose level, i.e., pancreatic ß-cell insulin delivery.

- **Implantable intraperitoneal delivery system:** A means of open-loop insulin delivery from a subcutaneously implanted computer-driven insulin reservoir surgically placed in the abdominal wall with a delivery line threaded into the peritoneal cavity.

- **Brittle diabetes:** A term that refers to diabetes manifested by recurrent episodes of ketosis or ketoacidosis and/or severe hypoglycemia that are significant enough to endanger life or result in an inability to maintain a normal lifestyle. There may be multiple causes.

- **Hypoglycemia unawareness:** The inability of a person with diabetes to know when their blood glucose has declined to a hazardously low level.

Rationale for and Physiological Basis of Intensive Diabetes Management

Highlights

Intensive Diabetes Management

Physiological Basis of Intensive Management Methods
Normal Fuel Metabolism
Regulation of Fuel Metabolism
Implications for Therapy

Highlights
Rationale for and Physiological Basis of Intensive Diabetes Management

- Technological advancements in diabetes care allow individuals with diabetes the potential of approaching normal glycemic control.

- Glycemic control that approaches the nondiabetic state postpones or slows the progression of the retinal, renal, and neurologic complications of diabetes.

- Intensive diabetes management has the goal of achieving euglycemia or near-normal glycemia. This mode of treatment is the preferred therapeutic approach for most patients with diabetes, whether they have insulin-dependent (type I) or non-insulin-dependent (type II) diabetes.

- Intensive diabetes management works by delivering insulin and adjusting factors such as diet and exercise to approximate normal fuel metabolism. Elements of this approach include
  - a relatively constant low blood insulin level during fasting
  - a rapid increase in blood insulin level after meals, in an amount appropriate to the amount of food eaten
  - a decrease in insulin levels with rigorous or prolonged exercise or prolonged fasting, and
  - frequent blood glucose testing to guide adjustments in insulin dose or other parts of the regimen.

Rationale for and Physiological Basis of Intensive Diabetes Management

For decades, the main goal of diabetes management has been to lower blood glucose levels and eradicate diabetic complications. The effectiveness of glycemic control in lessening the risk of microvascular and macrovascular complications was debated without consensus.

Advances made over the last 15 yr, such as self-monitoring of blood glucose, the measurement of glycated hemoglobin, and the availability of pure insulin preparations, created a technical basis for intensive diabetes management. Clinical studies in patients with insulin-dependent (type I) diabetes and in pregnant women with diabetes showed sufficient benefits to prompt a consensus on intensive diabetes management as a therapeutic standard of care. The Diabetes Control and Complications Trial showed without question that glycemic control that approaches the nondiabetic state postpones or slows the progression of the retinal, renal, and neurologic complications of diabetes. Other benefits include diminished risk to mother and fetus during pregnancy, minimized aberrations in lipoprotein metabolism, and normalized host-defense mechanisms (Table 1.1). An increased risk of hypoglycemic reactions, undesired weight gain, an altered quality of life made burdensome by the technical demands of intensified therapy, and greater personal expense in implementation were identified as risks of intensive management (Table 1.2). Successful application of this management strategy varies among patients.

Table 1.1. Benefits of Successful Intensive Diabetes Management

- A feeling of physical and emotional well-being and of "being in control"
- Lowered risk of microvascular complications developing and/or progressing
- Lowered maternal and fetal morbidity and or mortality during pregnancy
- Diminished risk of congenital malformations in the fetus
- Potential lowering of risk of macrovascular complications
- Optimal linear growth in children
- Greater freedom of lifestyle and daily schedule
- Greater knowledge and insight into diabetes care
- More predictable blood glucose values
- Better control of the dawn phenomenon

Table 1.2. Risks of Intensive Diabetes Management

- More frequent and potentially dangerous hypoglycemia
- If near-normal glycemia is goal, potential for hypoglycemia unawareness
- Perception of personal failure if unsuccessful in meeting goals
- Weight gain
- Diabetic ketoacidosis if using continuous subcutaneous insulin infusion
- Perception by the patient of more personal time spent caring for diabetes

INTENSIVE DIABETES MANAGEMENT

Intensive diabetes management is a mode of treatment that has the goal of achieving euglycemia or near-normal glycemia. Meeting this goal involves the integration of several diabetes treatment components into the individual's lifestyle. These components must include

- individualized medication regimen
- frequent blood glucose monitoring
- active adjustment of medication, food, and/or activity, based on blood glucose results
- use of blood glucose results to meet individually defined treatment goals
- ongoing interaction between the individual and the health-care team
  - assessment

Table 1.3. Indications for Intensive Diabetes Management

- Otherwise healthy adults with either type I or type II diabetes
- Purposeful therapeutic attempt to avoid or lessen microvascular complications
- All pregnant women with diabetes; all women with diabetes who plan a pregnancy
- Any person who wishes to achieve near-normal glycemic control
- Management of "brittle" diabetes
- Availability of experienced health-care professionals
- Selected adolescents and older children
- Patients who have had kidney transplantation for diabetic nephropathy

- education
- medical care and treatment
- emotional and psychological support
- frequent objective assessment of glycemic control (HbA_{1c}).

Table 1.4. Contraindications to Intensive Diabetes Management

- Short life expectancy
- Lack of desire by the patient to implement intensive diabetes management
- Social reasons
  - Inability to afford expenses of intensive diabetes management
  - Refusal to perform the technical tasks necessary for success and/or safety
  - Refusal to agree to scheduled follow-up visits
  - Inability to comprehend the techniques of implementation
- Presence of extensive end-stage microvascular complications
  - Blindness
  - Chronic, irremediable autonomic neuropathic complications
  - End-stage renal failure
- Infants and young children
- Active cardiovascular and/or cerebrovascular complications present
- Any medical, social, or psychological problem that negates risk-benefit ratio
- No experienced health-care professionals available

In addition, a thorough understanding of diabetes and its management by all involved in the daily care of this disease is crucial.

Intensive diabetes management is the preferred therapeutic approach for most patients with diabetes mellitus (Table 1.3). This position is based on the results of prospective studies that show that lowering mean blood glucose levels and glycated hemoglobin toward normal, over time, impedes the development or worsening of the microvascular complications of diabetes. Data are available for patients with type I diabetes and, because of the common basis of chronic hyperglycemia in the pathogenesis of these problems, are inferred for patients with non-insulin-dependent (type II) diabetes. Additionally, it is clear that intensive diabetes management in women who plan a pregnancy or who are pregnant lowers maternal morbidity and mortality to a level that matches the risk of women without diabetes. The fetus is protected from an adversarial maternal milieu by euglycemia; the risk of peripartum complications and congenital malformations closely approaches that of the offspring of a mother without diabetes.

Most patients with type I diabetes will require multiple daily insulin injections or an insulin pump to achieve the goals of treatment. For patients with type II diabetes, successful intensified therapy (with goals similar to those in type I diabetes) requires careful medical nutrition therapy and regular physical exercise. In patients with type II diabetes with greater degrees of insulin deficiency, supplemental oral antidiabetic agents, i.e., sulfonylureas or biguanides, and/or insulin will be needed to achieve near-normal glycemia. The goals of therapy may necessarily be modified in some patients because of age, comorbid states, ability of regular follow-up assessments, or other individual clinical situations that make the risks of intensified diabetes management greater than the benefits (Table 1.4).

The balance between risk and benefit is more delicate in the young child or the patient with type II diabetes than in younger, healthier patients with type I diabetes, where scientific data present a clear rationale for intensive therapy.

PHYSIOLOGICAL BASIS OF INTENSIVE MANAGEMENT METHODS

Intensive diabetes management is an attempt to normalize fuel metabolism by delivering insulin, and by manipulating or adjusting for other important factors, to approximate normal physiology. Although the goal of completely normal physiology cannot be met with available methods, it is possible to improve glycemic control enough to have dramatic impact on risk of chronic complications.

Normal Fuel Metabolism

Fuel metabolism is regulated by a complex system of
- multiple tissues and organs
- intracellular enzymatic systems to use nutrient fuels, and
- hormones and other factors to regulate the system to
  - distribute ingested nutrients to organs and tissues according to needs for mechanical or chemical work and tissue growth or renewal
  - provide for storage of excess nutrients as glycogen or fat, and
  - allow release of energy from storage depots as needed during periods of fasting or high energy use.

Carbohydrate metabolism. Carbohydrate in the form of glucose is a major energy source for muscle and the brain. The brain is nearly totally dependent on glucose, whereas muscle also uses fat for fuel. The two main sources of circulating glucose are hepatic glucose production and ingested carbohydrate. After absorption of the last meal is complete, glucose production by the liver must supply all the glucose needed for tissues that do not store glucose, such as the brain. This is referred to as basal glucose production and is generally ~2 mg · kg^{-1} body wt · min^{-1} in adults. About 75% of basal glucose production is from glycogenolysis; the rest is from gluconeogenesis.

Ingested carbohydrate is hydrolyzed into component sugars during gut absorption, producing a postprandial rise in blood glucose level that peaks 90–120 min after the meal. The magnitude and rate of rise in blood glucose is determined by many factors, including the size of the meal, the physical state of the food, e.g., solid, liquid, cooked, or raw, and the presence of other nutrients, e.g., fat and fiber slow down digestion. These factors usually have more effect on glycemia than the type of carbohydrate, i.e., "simple" or "complex." Identical quantities of simple and complex carbohydrate have been shown to affect blood glucose similarly.

Glucose is either oxidized for energy or stored as glycogen or fat. Sixty to seventy percent of an oral carbohydrate load is stored, mostly as glycogen; the remainder is oxidized for immediate energy needs.

Protein metabolism. Ingested protein is absorbed as amino acids that may be used in three ways
- synthesis of new protein,
- oxidation to provide energy, and
- conversion to glucose (gluconeogenesis).

During fasting, conversion of protein to glucose is an important means of maintaining blood glucose levels. Alanine is the major amino acid substrate for gluconeogenesis. Branched chain amino acids constitute a large fraction of ingested protein. They may be oxidized for energy, used for protein synthesis, or converted to alanine, which in turn can be converted to glucose.

Fat metabolism. Fat is the major form of stored energy. Fat stored as triglyceride is converted to free fatty acids plus glycerol by lipolysis. Free fatty acids from adipose tissue may be transported to muscle for oxidation. Oxidation of free fatty acids produces the ketone bodies acetoacetate and ß-hydroxybutyrate (referred to as ketogenesis). Ketone bodies are therefore a stage in fat oxidation and may be further metabolized as energy sources. Much of the ingested fat in a meal is efficiently stored in adipose tissue or muscle fat deposits. Only a small part of a glucose load is taken up by fat cells, although chronic nutritional excess obviously results in accumulation of stored fat, because ingested fat is not used and other excess nutrients (glucose) are used to synthesize fat.

Regulation of Fuel Metabolism

Fuel metabolism is regulated by several hormones. The CNS has an important role in this regulation, either through hormones or in other ways that are incompletely understood. The important hormones and their effects are summarized in Table 1.5 and discussed in more detail below.

Insulin. Insulin is the only hypoglycemic hormone. It acts by increasing glucose uptake for oxidation and storage and by decreasing glucose production. Insulin also inhibits lipolysis and thereby limits the availability of fatty acids for oxidation and limits ketogenesis.

Insulin is secreted in two major patterns.

- Basal secretion produces relatively constant, low insulin levels that act to restrain lipolysis and glucose production. Without the low levels of basal insulin secretion during fasting, glucose production, lipolysis, and ketogenesis increase substantially, causing hyperglycemia, hyperlipidemia, and ketosis. Insulin secretion falls during fasting and exercise, when tissues require access to stored energy. This allows increased glucose production and lipolysis, making stored energy available. Blood glucose level is the dominant stimulus for insulin secretion. ß-Cells of the pancreatic islet "monitor" glucose levels constantly so that insulin secretion is closely linked to changes in glycemia. Even small increases in blood glucose normally cause an increase in insulin secretion.
- Postprandial secretion increases rapidly to a level many times greater than basal secretion. Higher postprandial insulin levels turn off glucose production and lipolysis completely and stimulate uptake of ingested glucose by tissues.

Counterregulatory hormones. Glucagon, catecholamines (epinephrine and norepinephrine), cortisol, and growth hormone are termed counterregulatory hormones because they

Table 1.5. Regulation of Fuel Metabolism by Hormones

	INSULIN	GLUCAGON	CATECHOLAMINE	CORTISOL	GROWTH HORMONE
Glucose uptake	+	0	0	0	0
Gluconeogenesis	-	+	+	+	0
Glycogenolysis	-	+	+	+	+
Lipolysis	-	+	+	+	+
Ketogenesis	-	+	+	+	+

+, increases; -, decreases; 0, no effect.

generally have actions opposite to those of insulin. Each is produced under different circumstances, and has somewhat different effects on metabolism. Together with insulin, they regulate metabolism under widely varying conditions. These hormones are often referred to as stress hormones, because they increase in response to stress. It has been suggested that this response is designed to provide the extra energy often needed to deal with stress.

Glucagon is the first line of defense against hypoglycemia in people without diabetes. It rises rapidly when blood glucose levels fall, and stimulates hepatic glucose production. In type I diabetes, glucagon secretion in response to hypoglycemia is lost. This results in a loss of this important defense mechanism against hypoglycemia.

Catecholamines are produced at times of stress ("fight or flight") and also stimulate release of stored energy. They are the major defense against hypoglycemia. Hypglycemia unawareness and sluggish recovery from hypoglycemia may occur when this defense is defective. Patients with hypoglycemia un-awareness are at high risk for severe hypoglycemia and should intensify glucose control only with great caution.

Cortisol secretion also increases at times of stress. Its major effect is to stimulate gluconeogenesis. This effect is much slower than glucagon, however, so cortisol is not effective in protecting against acute hypoglycemia.

Growth hormone also has slow effects on glucose metabolism. A major surge of growth hormone secretion occurs during sleep and is responsible for a rise in blood glucose levels in the early morning, termed the *dawn phenomenon*. In normal physiology, a slight increase in insulin secretion compensates for the effects of growth hormone, but in diabetes the result may be variable morning hyperglycemia related to variable nocturnal growth hormone secretion.

Implications for Therapy

The most effective treatment regimens for diabetes will approximate normal physiology. Important elements of treatment include
- a relatively constant low blood insulin level during fasting
- a rapid increase in blood insulin level after meals, in an amount appropriate to the amount of food eaten
- a decrease in insulin levels with rigorous or prolonged exercise or prolonged fasting, and
- frequent blood glucose testing to guide adjustments in insulin dose and other parts of the regimen.

Even the most complicated insulin regimens cannot account for all the conditions that influence blood glucose levels. Therefore, the best methods available do not produce "perfect control"; there will be variations in blood glucose that are difficult or impossible to understand. In other words, patients with diabetes may follow through with every aspect of management and still have unexplained blood glucose variations. Nevertheless, attention to many small details greatly improves the control that can be achieved.

BIBLIOGRAPHY

Colwell JA: DCCT findings: applicability and implications for NIDDM. *Diabetes Rev* 2:277–91, 1994

Davidson MB: Why the DCCT applies to NIDDM patients. *Clin Diabetes* 12:141–44, 1994

DCCT Research Group: The effect of intensive treatment of diabetes on the development and progression of long-term complications in insulin-dependent diabetes mellitus. *N Engl J Med* 329:977–86, 1993

Genuth S: Insulin use in NIDDM. *Diabetes Care* 13:1240–64, 1990

Hirsch IB, Farkas-Hirsch R, Skyler JS: Intensive insulin therapy for treatment of type I diabetes. *Diabetes Care* 13:1265–83, 1990

Kitzmiller JL: Sweet success with diabetes: the development of insulin therapy and glycemic control for pregnancy. *Diabetes Care* 16 (Suppl. 3):107–21,1993

Lasker RD: The DCCT: implications for policy and practice. *N Engl J Med* 329:1035–36, 1993

Reicherd P, Nilsson B-Y, Rosenqvist U: The effect of long-term intensified insulin treatment on the development of microvascular complications of diabetes. *N Engl J Med* 329:304–309, 1993

Rosenzweig JL, Beaser R, Crowell S, Friedlander E, Ganda OP, Halford B, Jacobson A, Rand LI, Stewart C, Wolfsdorf JI: Findings of the Diabetes Control and Complications Trial. In *Joslin's Diabetes Mellitus*. 13th ed. Kahn CR, Weir GC, Eds. Philadelphia, PA, Lea & Febiger, 1994, p. 1022–27

Taylor R, Foster B, Kyne-Grzebalski M, Vanderpump M: Insulin regimens for the noninsulin dependent: impact on diurnal metabolic state and quality of life. *Diabetic Med* 11:551–57, 1994

Zinman B: Insulin regimens and strategies for IDDM. *Diabetes Care* 16 (Suppl. 3): 24–28, 1993

The Team Approach

Highlights

The Concept of Team Management

Integrated Diabetes Management Team

Role Definition

Team Communication

Functional Considerations

Highlights
The Team Approach

- Multidisciplinary team management is an effective and efficient alternative for the provision of the multidimensional care and support that is demanded by diabetes.

- Multidisciplinary team management provides the patient with
  - medical diagnosis and treatment
  - focused diabetes education
  - nutrition therapy and management assistance, and
  - psychosocial evaluation and support.

- Team management necessitates
  - identification of a common goal between team members
  - shared decision making
  - open communication and ongoing collaboration, and
  - active involvement by all team members.

- The treatment plan must be individualized and incorporate
  - medical priorities and concerns and
  - patient's abilities, willingness, and readiness.

- Intensive management of diabetes requires active participation by the patient and health-care providers.

- Active patient participation in care requires willingness to
  - become involved in daily self-care
  - acquire skills necessary to make reasoned decisions
  - define the daily schedule and environment
  - implement the necessary treatment interventions, and
  - maintain frequent, open, and honest communication with health-care providers.

- Effective treatment intervention
  - establishes treatment goals
  - negotiates needed lifestyle changes, and
  - facilitates achievement of knowledgeable independence in self-care.

- Effective team communication requires
  - common philosophy and message
  - common expectations
  - flexible professional boundaries
  - shared responsibility, and
  - open approach to management interventions.

- Patients must hear the same message from each member of the treatment team for any message to be heard.

The Team Approach

The American Diabetes Association (ADA) supports the position that intensive diabetes management should be considered for most patients with diabetes. Like many other chronic diseases, management of diabetes requires that lifestyle issues be addressed if the interventions are to be accepted and successfully integrated. However, few other disorders demand such a high level of daily attention to behavioral issues and choices. Although most health-care providers recognize the existence of these issues, objective analysis of current diabetes health-care practices reveals a significant discrepancy between this knowledge and actual practice patterns. This necessitates a reevaluation of all previous diabetes health-care delivery practices. The message "glycemic control matters" must now be translated into individually defined health-care choices and decisions.

Over the past decade, multidisciplinary team management has become increasingly accepted as an effective and efficient alternative for the provision of the multidimensional care and support that is demanded by diabetes. This approach emphasizes focused diabetes education, nutrition management, and psychosocial support. These complement the traditional medical model approach that includes medical diagnosis and treatment. Comprehensive diabetes management by a multidisciplinary team approach does not obviate the need for or value of the solo practitioner. Instead, it illustrates the unique nature of diabetes management. Time and multidimensional expertise are significant constraints in the health-care system that currently cares for most individuals with diabetes. In the presence of irrefutable data that intensive diabetes management is important, appropriate care can no longer occur in the context of three or four 15-min medical management visits per year.

THE CONCEPT OF TEAM MANAGEMENT

Multidisciplinary team management encompasses a group of individuals from various disciplines who are focused on common health-care goals. A team is a group of individuals with similar interests and different areas of professional expertise. As a group, they have a common purpose or focus. Each team member is responsible for contributing opinions and making decisions that support the common goals. The effectiveness of any team depends on the members' ability to communicate and collaborate in the identification and achievement of their goals (Table 2.1).

Management of diabetes necessitates active involvement by both patient and health-care providers. Once the commitment to care has been made, treatment plan definition can occur. Issues to consider when establishing a treatment plan are

- patient's understanding of diabetes treatment and management
- ongoing assessment and treatment based on medical diagnosis and needs
- acquisition of technical skills, knowledge, and proficiency
- ongoing assessment of the management components and treatment approach
- recognition of the obstacles to appropriate self-care, and development of intervention strategies to address them, and
- establishment of a means of communication that facilitates

Table 2.1. Factors That Influence Team Function

- Common goals and objectives of the team
- Role expectations of each team member
- Decision-making process
- Communication patterns
- Leadership
- Accepted practice behaviors for team members (informally defined)

Figure 2.1. Treatment Plan

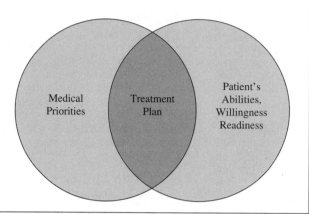

ongoing interaction between the patient and the health-care providers.

The treatment plan must be individualized to the patient, taking into consideration medical priorities and giving ample attention to the patient's abilities, as well as their willingness and readiness to carry through the defined interventions (Fig. 2.1). Knowledge of the need to make changes in one's health-care behavior is sometimes insufficient in motivating positive change. Thus, patient readiness must be a constant component of the treatment plan equation.

Figure 2.2. Integrated Diabetes Health-Care Team

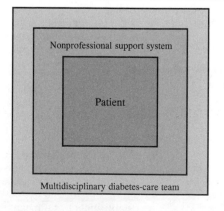

INTEGRATED DIABETES MANAGEMENT TEAM

The individual with diabetes is the central member of the diabetes health-care team and needs to be trained to assume most of the responsibility for ongoing care. This individual is guided in self-care practice and management interventions by the multidisciplinary health-care team. The patient's self-management efforts are supported further by nonprofessional individuals who play important roles in day-to-day life, such as spouses, parents, children, teachers, and coworkers. For this team to function effectively, each member must assume certain responsibilities (Fig. 2.2). Team effectiveness will determine the impact, both positive and negative, on patient care.

As the central member of this team, the patient must make the commitment to self-care (Table 2.2). Without this commitment, progress will be absent. Once made, this commitment is expanded to include a willingness to become an *active participant* in health care. Active participation means

- defining the environment in which the diabetes care will occur
- establishing the daily schedule
- implementing the necessary treatment interventions
- acquiring the necessary skills to make reasoned decisions regarding treatment plan changes, and
- being willing to maintain frequent, open, and honest communication with the health-care team.

Ongoing care involves the integration of complex self-care techniques and subsequent alterations of lifestyle habits and patterns. Once integrated, patients are afforded increased flexibility in the management regimen and an increased sense of mastery and control over their disease.

Health-care providers have the responsibility to work with the patient to establish treatment goals and, then, to negotiate needed lifestyle changes (Table 2.3). The goal of intervention is to facilitate the achievement of knowledgeable independence in self-care, based on the individual's abilities.

Ongoing communication for problem-solving, feedback, and reality-based reinforcement guides the patient's efforts.

The health-care team plays a vital role in the implementation of intensive diabetes management (Table 2.4). However, before assisting patients with treatment plan implementation, health-care providers must be realistic about their personal beliefs regarding the value of intensive diabetes treatment. Unless providers are knowledgeable *and* committed to the concept of intensive management and have access to the additional resources needed to ensure safe and effective treatment, their ability to assist patients in defining and/or achieving intensive treatment goals will be compromised. Patient education programs must incorporate

- technical skills training
- adjustment guidelines for variable diet, exercise, and current glycemia
- problem-solving techniques, and
- risk management guidance.

All team members must have a broad understanding of diabetes and its management. Health-care providers must also ensure that ADA's Clinical Practice Recommendations are met (see BIBLI-OGRAPHY). Achieving this goal necessitates an awareness and use of the Clinical Practice Recommendations to define practice behaviors and health-care delivery.

The availability of 24-h access to health-care providers who are knowledgeable in intensive diabetes self-management often can avert trips to emergency rooms and can prevent hospitalizations. If such provider availability does not exist, the risks associated with intensive management may outweigh the potential benefits and, thus, interfere with a patient's willingness to participate in these efforts.

If the health-care team is not readily available or adequately prepared with the additional knowledge, skills, and resources necessary to implement intensive diabetes management and/or is not committed to the concept of this form of therapy, it may be better to refer those patients who wish to intensify their management to centers that are prepared to undertake this endeavor. A collaborative relationship between the personnel at these referral centers and the primary care provider is crucial to the success and effectiveness of the treatment plan. This is particularly important in view of the fact that the primary care provider is often the recipient of after-hours calls from patients.

Table 2.2. Patient Responsibilities

- *Commit to self-care*
- Participate as active member of treatment team
- Make ongoing decisions regarding daily management
- Identify environmental factors impacting plan
- Communicate frequently and honestly with diabetes-care team

---

Table 2.3. Health-Care Provider Responsibilities

- Know ADA's Clinical Practice Recommendations
- Understand the scientific and clinical data on which ADA's Clinical Practice Recommendations are based
- Use ADA's Clinical Practice Recommendations to define and evaluate diabetes-care delivery and practices
- Facilitate implementation of the treatment plan through ongoing education and communication
- Foster the development of "knowledgeable independence" in self-care practices
- Provide feedback and reinforcement
- Provide access to health-care providers who are experienced in diabetes self-management and supportive of guided self-management

---

Table 2.4. Health-Care Team Characteristics That Influence Success of Intensive Diabetes Management Efforts

- Belief in the benefits of intensive diabetes management
- Appreciation for the value of patient autonomy in self-care
- Willingness to commit resources and efforts to intensive management implementation
- Ability to provide or to access multidisciplinary education and health-care expertise
- Understanding of the risks associated with intensive diabetes management
- Availability of 24-h assistance in problem solving

ROLE DEFINITION

A clear understanding of the team goals, as well as individual member roles and responsibilities, is a key requirement for a team to be successful. Each member's contribution to the team effort should be determined by their educational background, degrees/credentials, individual abilities, experience, interests, and overall goals of team operation. Typical roles and/or responsibilities for the physician, nurse, dietitian, and mental health professional members of the diabetes-care team are listed in Table 2.5. Note that there

---

Table 2.5. Typical Roles and Responsibilities of the Diabetes-Care Team Members

- **Role of physician**
    - Establish medical diagnosis and define treatment
    - Provide rationale for treatment
    - Collaborate with the patient and team to design and implement a treatment plan
    - Encourage the patient to work with the team to design and implement a treatment plan
    - Oversee total patient management

- **Role of nurse manager/educator/clinician**
    - Self-care assessment
    - Patient education: self-management skills, technical proficiency, compensatory adjustments, problem solving
    - Family education/assessment
    - Interim contact: acute problem management, preventive education, blood glucose pattern review
    - Team effort coordination

- **Role of dietitian**
    - Nutrition assessment
    - Meal plan development
    - Specialized medical nutrition therapy
    - Interim contact: meal plan integration/modification, compensatory adjustments for variable food intake and/or exercise, blood glucose pattern review

- **Role of mental health professional**
    - Elicit and address patient/family concerns and fears
    - Identify treatment obstacles
    - Provide patient/family support
    - Provide team support

is considerable overlap between roles and that few roles are exclusive.

The team's effectiveness will be influenced by the ability of its members to collaborate, rather than to compete. Within the multidisciplinary framework, no team member operates in isolation. Instead, expertise and strengths are combined to enhance the delivery of comprehensive patient care. The addition of these disciplines to the current medical model serves to extend the scope and availability of assessment, intervention, follow-up, and treatment for the individual with diabetes.

Comprehensive team management also can occur in settings where, through referral, a team has been built of members located at different sites or within separate facilities. For this approach to be effective, added emphasis must be placed on ongoing, accurate, and complete communication between the team members involved. Creativity and ingenuity can be employed to facilitate the communication process using fax, e-mail, and modem transmissions, as well as verbal and written communication. Absence of all team members within a given facility should not be a deterrent to the use of a multidisciplinary approach to diabetes management.

In practice, settings where a full complement of team members is not available and referral to a tertiary care center is unacceptable, attempts still must be made to provide comprehensive education and care. The ability of a modified team to safely and successfully implement intensive management will depend on the abilities and capabilities of the professionals involved.

TEAM COMMUNICATION

Integrated team functioning requires the definition of a common philosophy regarding diabetes-care practices and the development of a consistent treatment message and approach (Table 2.6). Patients must hear the same message from all members of the treatment team for any message to be heard. Conflicting or incongruent directives from providers interfere with the

Table 2.6. Team Communication

- Common philosophy and message
- Common expectations
- Flexible professional boundaries
- Shared responsibility
- Open approach to management interventions

patient's willingness and/or ability to carry out the treatment recommendations.

Within treatment teams, role definitions and boundaries serve to define certain tasks. However, the complex nature of diabetes necessitates flexibility in these boundaries, resulting in a blending of roles and sharing of responsibilities. By maintaining openness regarding the interdependent working possibilities between team members, patients are more likely to receive comprehensive care. Rigid boundaries surrounding professional disciplines often result in a territorial approach to patient care, which limits the team's ability to meet the patient's needs whenever any team member is absent.

Team meetings provide an opportunity for members to readily communicate with each other and to maintain a focused approach to their health-care practices (Table 2.7). If held on a regular basis, team meetings facilitate review of individual patient problems and/or progress, facilitate identification of clinic problems and patient care trends, and provide the forum for active problem-solving sessions. In this context, problem solving and solution definition take on a multidisciplinary flavor, decreasing the chance for con-

Table 2.7. Team Meetings

- Maintain focus on common philosophy and goals
- Review patient progress and/or problems
- Identify system or clinic trends
- Provide active, multidisciplinary problem solving and solution definition
- Establish intrateam support

flicts between the members of the treatment team. Team meetings also facilitate ongoing support between the health-care providers, with the mental health professional often assisting other staff members in recognizing behaviors or intervention styles that may be counterproductive to the achievement of treatment goals. In the absence of regularly scheduled team meetings, an alternative communication strategy between team members needs to be identified (i.e., e-mail, voice mail, or fax) to ensure that patient care is comprehensive and that the messages received by patients are consistent.

FUNCTIONAL CONSIDERATIONS

Team management may necessitate a functional change in the hierarchy of patient care responsibility. Team members who are certified as diabetes educators (CDEs) by the National Certification Board for Diabetes Educators are expected to function at a specialist level. Certification provides an objective means of defining and evaluating practice behaviors. As certified practitioners, these health-care professionals assume a portion of the legal responsibility for education practices and diabetes-care delivery. In addition, the establishment of National Standards for Diabetes Self-Management Education Programs by the diabetes community, which are used in ADA's Recognition Program to identify quality diabetes education programs, has further defined the level of intervention and care expected of these practitioners and the programs they administer.

Team management, while still being viewed as more innovative than customary, represents a situation where practices and/or procedures, formerly performed by the physician, become a routine and accepted part of the non-physician provider's role. Acceptance of this expanded role brings the expectation that practitioners will be responsible, at least in part, for treatment direction, decisions, and interventions. The conduct of these activities is guided by written standardized procedures and educational interventions with stated goals, objectives, and content.

BIBLIOGRAPHY

American Diabetes Association: *Clinical Practice Recommendations 1995. Diabetes Care* 18 (Suppl. 1):1–96, 1995

American Diabetes Association position statement: Standards of medical care for patients with diabetes mellitus. *Diabetes Care* 17: 616–23, 1994

DCCT Study Group: The effect of intensive treatment of diabetes on the development and progression of long-term complications in insulin dependent diabetes mellitus. *N Engl J Med* 329:977–86, 1993

Etzwiler DD: Primary-care teams and a systems approach to diabetes management. *Clin Diabetes* 12: 50–52, 1994

Flavin K, White NH: The intensive insulin therapy team. *Diabetes Educator* 15:249–52, 1989

Franz MJ, Callahan T, Castle G: Changing roles: educators and clinicians. *Clin Diabetes* 12: 53–54, 1994

Lorber DL, Lagana DJ: The health-care team in diabetes. *Prac Diabetol* 10:15–21, 1991

Lowe JI, Herranen M: Conflict in teamwork: understanding roles and relationships. *Soc Work Health Care* 3:323–30, 1978

Palmer LI: Ethical and legal implications of diabetes self-management. *Prac Diabetol* 8:1–4, 1989

Ratner RE, El-Gamassy ER: Legal aspects of the team approach to diabetes treatment. *Diabetes Educator* 16:113–16, 1990

Yale University DCCT Group: Weekly meetings focus team efforts. *Diabetes Spectrum* 7:77–78, 1994

Diabetes Self-Management Education

Highlights

Integration of the Team Approach

Diabetes Continuing Education

Assessment

Instruction
> Environment
> Planning
> Content
> Sequencing of Classes
> Approaches/Strategies

Motivation

Negotiation

Evaluation

Documentation

Highlights
Diabetes Self-Management
Education

- The patient using intensive diabetes management must translate new information and skills into behavior change. Each interaction with the patient is an opportunity for the health-care provider to teach and encourage. The team approach is best exemplified when information is consistent among team members.

- The patient's readiness to learn new information is a necessary component of any negotiated education plan. The individual will be most receptive when the education is salient to his or her current needs. In addition, eliciting the patient's commitment to behavior change is another integral component of any education program.

- Educational assessment includes information about the patient's knowledge, skills, attitudes, and current diabetes-care behaviors. The patient must possess a basic level of understanding before learning the more sophisticated aspects of intensive diabetes self-management.

- Education is communication and requires careful planning, with delivery of pertinent information. Classes should be sequenced to build on existing knowledge. Teaching methods include the use of print and audiovisual materials. These items must be content appropriate, readable, and culturally sensitive.

- Intensive diabetes management requires active patient involvement. As part of their education, some individuals may need assistance in actively participating in their care.

- Evaluating the success of patient education can be practical and quick. By using a series of "what if" questions, the educator is able to assess the patient's problem-solving abilities.

- Recording key aspects of the education experience allows the diabetes educators to share information with primary care and referring physicians.

Diabetes Self-Management Education

As the Diabetes Control and Complications Trial (DCCT) demonstrated, diabetes self-management education is integral to the success of an intensive management program. The patient embarking on the road to tight control must not only understand the complexities of diabetes and perform the technical skills necessary but also must believe in the management strategies and in himself or herself. Intensive management requires the patient to assume an active role in clinical decisions on a daily basis. To do this safely and effectively, the patient needs a supportive, knowledgeable, and accessible professional health-care team.

Diabetes self-management training is successful when the patient is able to translate the information and skill behavior change. Consequently, diabetes education is more than a lecture or two on how to control the disease. Instead, it is an ongoing program of assessment, instruction, motivation, negotiation, and evaluation delivered by a team of diabetes professionals.

INTEGRATION OF THE TEAM APPROACH

A coordinated team of professionals provides depth to the patient's diabetes self-management education. The physician, nurse manager/educator/ clinician, dietitian, and mental health professional, as well as the pharmacist and exercise physiologist, all contribute unique skills and focus. The physician may create a team by referring to a community-based patient education program or to local diabetes educators. The American Diabetes Association maintains a list of nationally recognized education programs. The American Association of Diabetes Educators keeps a roster of certified diabetes educators.

Diabetes education should never stand alone. Instead, it is a component of the care and management for the patient with diabetes. All members of the treatment team are teachers. Each contact with the patient is an opportunity to teach or evaluate the effect of teaching.

Information must be consistent across professionals. This allows the patient to develop the necessary trust in the management plan and in the health-care providers. Educational materials must also be consistent in content. Consequently, each team member should know what the others are teaching.

DIABETES CONTINUING EDUCATION

Diabetes information should be taught with the understanding that the subject requires a continual process of learning and adjusting. One class, or a series of classes, at diagnosis does not confer lifelong immunity! Instead, education should be viewed as a treatment that requires periodic boosters.

Patients vary in their willingness or readiness to learn. There are times when learner readiness is high: when new research findings are released, when new medications are available, when complications occur, and when developmental changes arise. These are times for the educator to capitalize on the patient's increased motivation.

ASSESSMENT

The first step in developing an individualized education plan is to gather information about the patient's current knowledge, skills, attitudes, and behaviors.

Because intensive management is so dependent on the patient's involvement and decision making, certain basic facts and skills are necessary. Table 3.1 lists the *entry-level* information for patients entering an intensive management program. In addition to information, the patient must accurately and safely perform certain self-management skills. These skills include

■ using a blood glucose meter

Table 3.1. Basic Facts for the Candidate for Intensive Diabetes Management

- Insulin action/insulin regimens
- Rationale for self-monitoring of blood glucose: testing frequency, goals, patterns
- Glycated hemoglobin: testing frequency, goals
- Nutrition management
  - Healthy food choices
  - Role of major nutrients: effect on blood glucose levels
  - Sick day management
  - Label reading
  - Dining out/convenience foods
- Effect of exercise
- Interaction of exercise, diet, and medication
- Hypoglycemia: causes, treatment, prevention
- Glucagon
- Identifying the dawn phenomenon
- Hyperglycemia: causes, treatment, prevention
- Ketoacidosis: causes, treatment, prevention
- Complications: causes, symptoms, prevention, monitoring
- Effect of daily living on diabetes control
  - Alcohol and other drugs/drug interactions
  - Tobacco
  - Work schedules
  - Traveling
  - Illness/medications and control
- Individual's evaluation of his/her efforts

  - troubleshooting problems with testing
  - testing urine ketones
  - record keeping
  - preparing and injecting insulin, and
  - caring for the feet.
  A careful educational assessment

Table 3.2. Eliciting the Patient's Beliefs

- What has been your experience with chronic health problems?
- How do you usually deal with success and failure?
- How has your diabetes affected your family?
- What worries or concerns you most about having diabetes?
- How do you typically learn new things?
- What one thing would you tell someone newly diagnosed with diabetes?
- What is the hardest part of diabetes management?

includes
- Personal and socioeconomic information: age; developmental level; level of education; family composition; significant others; cultural, religious, and ethnic factors; resources; insurance; and transportation.
- Diabetes information: type and duration of diabetes, current management approaches, previous management approaches, acute and chronic complications, previous diabetes education, and successes and problems with adherence.
- Other medical information: height, weight, blood pressure, pertinent laboratory values (e.g., blood glucose, glycated hemoglobin, lipids, and albumin), other illnesses, other medications, general health status, visual and hearing acuity, and motor skills.
- Lifestyle factors: use of alcohol, tobacco, or other social drugs; physical activity; stressors; occupation; recreation; and social support systems.
- Nutrition information: meal and snack times, locations, and typical foods; food preferences and intolerances; previous experience with "diets"; and previous nutrition education.
- Education factors: learning style, literacy, readiness to learn, decision-making skills, health beliefs (e.g., locus of control, confidence, experience with other chronic illnesses, coping patterns, fears, and concerns; Table 3.2), ability/willingness to seek help, expectations and capacity to deal with failure, assertiveness skills, organizational skills, response to an education plan, and motivators.

INSTRUCTION

Environment

The learning environment includes not just the physical facility, but also characteristics of the instructor who facilitates the learning. To help the patient focus on the content, the location should be quiet and free from distractions. Qualities of the teacher that promote learning are included in Table 3.3.

The educator must draw from an extensive knowledge base while translating this knowledge into language understandable to the learner/patient. Furthermore, the educator must be able to adjust an educational agenda to meet the learner's needs. For example, the educator may have determined that the patient should hear about different insulin programs, whereas the patient may want to learn about counting carbohydrates.

Education is a process of communication and reception of information. Throughout the education session, the educator assesses the learner's understanding. By asking the patient to restate the information or to use the information to solve a problem, the educator is able to evaluate learning.

Planning

As the assessment proceeds, the educator will identify topics and teaching approaches that are most appropriate for the patient. Shared goal setting is important. The plan for the education program becomes a negotiation between the teacher and learner. Although it is the educator's responsibility to identify knowledge deficits, it is the learner's job to provide an accurate medical and educational history and to acknowledge what must be learned to undertake intensive management safely.

Often, the patient *doesn't know what he needs to know* and may, in fact, be resistant to new information. Then, the educator's job is to gently challenge the patient's knowledge while presenting new information. The educator may need to remind the patient that medical knowledge about diabetes changes rapidly, and old information is being replaced with new ways of handling the disease.

Content

Topics especially pertinent for the patient implementing intensive diabetes management include
- nutritional guidelines and the effect of food on glycemic control
- insulin action and dosage adjustment
- exercise
- monitoring
- management of acute complications
- prevention and detection of chronic complications, and
- behavior change strategies.

A comprehensive curriculum list is included in Table 3.4.

Sequencing of Classes

There is far too much information to receive in one sitting. Effective diabetes education occurs over several contacts with the patient. The most meaningful education sessions build on the patient's existing knowledge and on content from previous sessions. For instance, one session may be spent discussing insulin regimens, the interpretation of blood glucose results, and record keeping. The next session may be spent reviewing blood glucose records and discussing and demonstrating insulin-adjustment techniques.

Table 3.3. Qualities of the Teacher

- Knowledge base is current and extensive
- Personal belief that patients can learn
- Empathy
- Genuineness
- Adaptable: has a variety of teaching approaches
- Sense of humor
- Ability to
  - Individualize information
  - Encourage questions
  - Allow adequate time for patient to answer
  - Use clear, simple, concrete explanations
  - Sequence educational topics
  - Involve others as needed
  - Repeat and reinforce facts
  - Evaluate understanding
  - Provide feedback

Table 3.4. Curriculum for Intensive Management

- Diabetes overview
  - DCCT results: long-term control and benefits
  - Benefits, risks, and management options for improving glucose control
- Stress and psychosocial adjustment
  - Effect of stress on control
  - Identifying stressors
  - Anticipating stress
  - Stress-management techniques
- Family involvement and social support
  - Sharing diabetes care: when and how
  - Seeking help
  - Support groups
  - Volunteer work
- Nutrition
  - Role of nutrients
  - Glycemic impact
  - Label reading
  - Carbohydrate counting/exchange systems/other
  - Alcohol: effect and use
  - Dining out
  - Evaluating effect of food adjust-ments/changes
- Exercise and activity
  - Effect of exercise
  - Exercise physiology
  - Prolonged effect, late postexercise hypoglycemia
  - Planning preexercise food
  - Evaluating effect of exercise
- Medications: insulin
  - Injection site selection
  - Insulin storage
  - Insulin preparation
  - Injection technique
  - Alternative delivery systems: cartridge systems and pumps
  - Insulin dose changes
    - Basal changes
    - Bolus changes (i.e., algorithms)
    - Pattern control
    - Evaluating effect of dose adjustment
    - When to call a physician or nurse
- Monitoring and use of results
  - Blood glucose meter use
    - Technique
    - Care of meter
    - Troubleshooting
- Fingerstick technique, care of skin
- Record keeping
- Understanding and using blood glucose results
- Testing at unusual times to gather information
- When to test urine ketones and interpretation of results
- Relationships among nutrition, exercise, medication, and blood glucose levels
  - Effect of daily variability
  - Effect of unusual days
    - Travel
    - Varying work schedules
  - Anticipating changes and making adjustments
- Prevention, detection, and treatment of acute complications
  - Identifying symptoms of hypo-glycemia
  - How symptoms may change as control tightens
  - Glucagon: who to train, precautions
  - Dawn phenomenon: recognizing and managing
  - Symptoms of hyperglycemia and its management
  - Diabetic ketoacidosis
- Prevention, detection, and treatment of chronic complications
  - Detection of problems
  - Routine health follow-up
  - Diabetes follow-up
  - Effect of intensification on existing complications
- Foot, skin, and dental care
  - Injection sites: more frequent injections
  - Prevention of infections
  - Dental prophylaxis
- Behavior change strategies, goal setting, risk factor reduction, and problem solving
  - Decision-making skills
  - Problem-solving approach
- Preconception, pregnancy, and postpartum management
- Use of health-care systems and community resources
  - Creating a diabetes management team
  - Financial impact and cost-saving strategies

Approaches/Strategies

Adults learn best when the information is immediately useful and salient. Thus, teaching a patient to implement an intensive management plan must include enough time to practice the decision making required and focus on information needed to implement the treatment plan. For example, if the patient will be using an algorithm to adjust insulin doses, then the educator must plan for opportunities to practice using that algorithm.

The educator should have a repertoire of *real life* examples to use when teaching. Most individuals will need help in developing the judgment and problem solving needed to make diabetes decisions. Consider, for instance, what a patient must evaluate in choosing an insulin dose before a meal. How much carbohydrate will be consumed? What is the current blood glucose? What range of insulin doses tends to work for this mealtime? What will the exercise level be in the next couple of hours? How long should the time between injection and meal be? Working through several examples with the patient allows the educator to model decision making. Decision making and problem solving are skills acquired and improved through practice alone. Mistakes are part of the learning process. The educator must create opportunity for practice and an environment where errors and misjudgments are used to learn, not criticize.

Other approaches include using print and audiovisual materials. Many excellent materials are available from commercial diabetes supply manufacturers. However, they must be individually evaluated for appropriate content, readability, and cultural sensitivity. Interactive educational materials, such as computer programs, food models, self-instructional materials, and games, add variety to the education program. Body Link from Boehringer-Mannheim, for instance, is a teaching tool that visually displays the complex pathophysiology of diabetes. A sample patient education handout is provided in Table 3.5.

Regardless of the methodology for instruction, one of the most effective approaches to encourage adherence is simple: Provide the literate patient with clear, written instructions! Patients generally remember very little from their time with the physician or educator. Written instructions can be the educator's most practical tool.

MOTIVATION

The process of patient education is intimately connected to behavior change. How the patient will use the information should be assessed by the educator. Simply asking the patient, "How will you try this at home?" or "What things will be easy/hard to do?" will often alert the educator to potential difficulties in adherence. Some questions to elicit the patient's commitment to behavior change are listed in Table 3.6.

NEGOTIATION

Some patients have adequate diabetes knowledge and wish to participate in their care, but lack the assertive communication or negotiation skills needed. They may feel intimidated by the health-care professional or by the system. Yet, patient involvement in treatment decisions is important for the individual on an intensive management program. So much of the daily management will be directed by the patient that his or her commitment to the plan is essential.

The educator may find that the patient actually needs assistance in communicating his or her needs to the physician. The patient's education plan may include tips on how to participate actively in the treatment plan.

EVALUATION

Often in a busy practice, patient education amounts to nothing more than the professional relaying information, with very little time directed at assessing how the information was received and implemented. Whether provided in the physician's office or in a formal classroom education setting, evaluat-

Table 3.5. Sample Worksheet for Intensive Diabetes Management

- **Goals for intensive blood glucose control**

Time of day	**ADA guidelines**	**Personal goals**
Fasting blood sugar	80–120 mg/dl	_____
Before meal	80–120 mg/dl	_____
Bedtime	100–140 mg/dl	_____
Average	110–150 mg/dl	_____

- **Goals for glycated hemoglobin**

	ADA guidelines	**Personal goals**
HbA_{1c}	6.0–7.0%	_____
HbA_1	7.0–9.0%	_____

- **Basal insulin**

Time	**Type**	**Dose**
_____	_____	_____
_____	_____	_____
_____	_____	_____

- **Bolus insulin**

Time	**Type**	**Dose**	**Carbohydrate amount**
_____	_____	_____	_____
_____	_____	_____	_____
_____	_____	_____	_____

ing the success of patient education can be quick and easy.

Tests and quizzes have a place in some education programs. However, for an adult learner, information that is useable will be remembered. Using a series of "what if" questions allows the educator to not only assess knowledge level but also to determine problem-solving abilities. A sample of such questions is provided in Table 3.7.

DOCUMENTATION

The diabetes educator is obligated to completely document the education process from assessment to evaluation. Checklists and documentation forms may be created to assist the educator in this task. Sample forms are provided in *Meeting the Standards: A Manual for Completing the American Diabetes Association Application for Recognition*. In addition to documenting the medical record, the educator should

Table 3.6. Verifying the Patient's Commitment

- How effective do you think this treatment will be for you?
- What part of the plan may be hard for you?
- Are you concerned about the time or expense?
- How will you know if the plan is working?
- How certain are you that you can do this?
- If now is not the right time for you to begin, when will the time be right?

also provide follow-up information to the referring physician. This provides continuity and consistency and facilitates the team approach.

CONCLUSION

Patient education is integral to the success of intensifying the individual's diabetes management. The patient must be skilled and knowledgeable to participate fully and daily in the necessary decisions about self-care. The physician, diabetes educators, and other professionals must form a unified teaching team to assure that the patient has consistent and accurate information. Providing diabetes self-management education requires attention to patient assessment, individualized instruction, and evaluation of patient response.

Table 3.7. Evaluating Learning and Problem Solving

- What would you do if
    - You had given yourself insulin and your restaurant meal was late?
    - You are supposed to take regular insulin before a meal, but your blood glucose level is 40 mg/dl?
    - You were planning to play tennis one hour after lunch?
    - You awakened with nausea and did not feel like eating?
    - Your blood glucose results did not coincide with how you felt?
- How would you adjust your insulin for extra food or exercise?
- What would you say to your doctor if you thought that the plan was not working?
- How will you adjust your management plan for special occasions and parties?

BIBLIOGRAPHY

Abouriz N, O'Connor P, Crabtree B, Schnatz JD: An outpatient model of integrated diabetes treatment and education: functional, metabolic, and knowledge outcomes. *Diabetes Educator* 20:416-21, 1994

American Diabetes Association: *Medical Management of Insulin-Dependent (Type I) Diabetes.* 2nd ed. Santiago JV, Ed. Alexandria, VA, Am. Diabetes Assoc., 1994

American Diabetes Association: *Meeting the Standards: A Manual for Completing the American Diabetes Association Application for Recognition.* 4th ed. Alexandria, VA, Am. Diabetes Assoc., 1995

Anderson L, Jenkins C (Eds.): Educational innovations in diabetes: where are we now? *Diabetes Spectrum* 7:89-124, 1994

Coonrod BA, Harris M, Betschart J: Frequency and determinants of diabetes patient education among adults in the U.S. population. *Diabetes Care* 17:852-58, 1994

DCCT Research Group: The impact of the trial coordinator in the Diabetes Control and Complications Trial (DCCT). *Diabetes Educator* 19:509-12, 1993

Farkas-Hirsch R, Hirsch I: The question is answered. now what? *Diabetes Care* 17:237-38, 1994

Haire-Joshu D: Promoting behavior change: teaching-learning strategies. In *Management of Diabetes Mellitus: Perspectives Across the Lifespan.* Haire-Joshu D, Ed. St. Louis, MO, Mosby, 1992, p. 556-90

Meichenbaum D, Turk D: *Facilitating Treatment Adherence.* New York, Plenum, 1987

Peragallo-Dittko V (Ed.): *A Core Curriculum for Diabetes Education.* 2nd ed. Chicago, IL, Am. Assoc. Diabetes Educators, 1993

Peyrot M, Rubin R: Modeling the effect of diabetes education on glycemic control. *Diabetes Educator* 20:143-148, 1994

Pichert J, Smeltzer C, Snyder G, Gregory R, Smeltzer R, Kinzer C: Traditional vs. anchored instruction for diabetes-related nutritional knowledge, skills, and behavior. *Diabetes Educator* 20:45-48, 1994

Rubin R, Peyrot M, Suadek C: Effect of diabetes education on self care, metabolic control, and emotional well-being. *Diabetes Care* 12:673-79, 1989

Schreiner B: Role of education in management. In *Diabetes Mellitus in Children and Adolescents*. Travis L, Brouhard B, Schreiner B, Eds. Philadelphia, PA, Saunders, 1987

Psychosocial Issues

Highlights

Assessing Patient Suitability for Intensification

Practicing Behavior
Assessing Psychosocial Status

Assessing the Effect of Stress on Glycemic Control

Assessing Coping Skills

Assessment of Diabetes-Related Coping
Identifying Psychosocial Resources

Helping Patients Deal With Complications

Helping Patients With Long-Term Adherence

Supporting Patients' Behavior Changes

Highlights
Psychosocial Issues

- Patients and their support people should be empowered, educated, and willing to accept responsibility for the increased self-care behaviors required by intensive diabetes management. Patient success with self-care behaviors and willingness to collaborate in treatment decisions are good indicators of future success with an intensive management plan.

- Before intensification of diabetes management begins,
  - patient self-management skills should be evaluated and training provided regarding skill deficits to establish competence with self-care and
  - medical or psychological conditions that impair a patient's ability to make, evaluate, or communicate treatment decisions should be identified so that the necessary psychosocial supports and safeguards can be put in place.

- The contribution of stress to glycemic status requires the evaluation of the patient's glycemic response and coping mechanisms. Stressful lifestyles do not preclude intensive management. However, each patient should be monitored for signs of depression and eating disorders so that resultant nonadherence with the treatment plan can be avoided and assure the patient's safety.

- The patient's emotional response to and attitudes toward complications should help shape the goals of management. Presence of complications need not deter patients from attempting to improve their glucose control. However, health-care providers need to help patients modify goals of treatment if complications associated with intensive diabetes management, e.g., worsening retinopathy, weight gain, and severe hypoglycemia, occur.

- Patients are more likely to succeed with self-care regimens that are responsive to lifestyle needs and do not present an overwhelming burden. To support behavior change, self-care behaviors should be taught, monitored for effectiveness, and modified in an ongoing fashion. However, lapses in self-care behaviors should be expected as a routine part of care.

- Psychosocial support is crucial to success with intensive diabetes management and must be ongoing. Support can come from health-care providers, family members, and diabetes-specific or community support groups.

Psychosocial Issues

Use of intensive management during the Diabetes Control and Complications Trial (DCCT) has taught us that patients can and will follow a medical regimen that is significantly more complex than that usually prescribed to treat diabetes. We also learned that if multidisciplinary services are available and user friendly, a high degree of compliance with a complex medical regimen can be achieved and there is a greater likelihood that treatment goals can be met without detrimental effects to the patient's quality of life. However, before intensification of diabetes management begins, it is important to identify which nonmedical or psychosocial factors promote or interfere with achieving good control and how intensive management will impact the patient's quality of life and psychosocial well-being. If intensive diabetes management affects the patient's job or school performance, interpersonal relationships, and emotional well-being in a negative manner, noncompliance with the prescribed regimen is likely, as is poorer glycemic control.

ASSESSING PATIENT SUITABILITY FOR INTENSIFICATION

Many patients come to the health-care provider with the stated goal of "improving their blood sugar control." However, emotional factors; lifestyle or financial barriers; and lack of, outdated, or inaccurate information may make immediate initiation of intensive management unfeasible. Instead, patients can be offered the option of intensifying self-care gradually. Self-management skills that fit their lifestyle and do not place an unmanageable burden on their daily routine can be added one at a time to the self-care routine.

Practicing Behavior

A technique commonly used in screen-ing patients for clinical trials—in which compliance is essential to answer the proposed question—is to ask candidates to maintain those self-care behaviors that approximate the experimental protocol for some period of time and assess their attitudes about and willingness to carry out the required behaviors. This technique is known as *prerandomization compliance screening*. It helps health-care providers assess the likely performance or compliance with behaviors that will be required during the course of the trial and the patient's willingness to follow regimen prescriptions. A patient's intention to continue to perform new self-care behaviors will also become evident. This technique allows patients to practice and become proficient in the desired self-care behaviors.

Compliance screening can easily be carried out in clinical practice. Compliance screening involves

- Assessment (with a questionnaire or interview format) of
  - the burden on the patient of self-care tasks: what is it like to live with the required tasks on a daily basis?
  - intentions regarding self-care behavior: does the patient intend to continue these tasks in the future?
  - attitudes about treatment prescriptions: does this method of treatment address the patients goals for diabetes care?
- Questioning of the patient regarding whether he or she
  - feels able and is willing to follow regimen changes
  - believes the changes will have positive impact on his or her health, and
  - believes the change in self-care tasks will not present an unmanageable lifestyle burden.
- Identifying gaps in the patient's knowledge, skills, and confidence so they can be addressed as part of the intervention process.
- Allowing the patient to try out and

become proficient in different treatment methods.

Because there is no one right way to treat diabetes, this approach allows patients to "try on" different treatment methods without concern of failure and provides a frame of reference wherein health-care providers do not label lack of success as noncompliance. Compliance screening provides the practitioner with the opportunity to assess and develop the cooperation and skills of the patient and develop the "best fit" treatment regimen.

A good use of compliance screening is in the selection of patients for insulin pump use. The pump can work well for those individuals who wish to achieve tight control but whose daily schedule does not fit easily into a routine. The pump provides the patient with the greatest freedom of lifestyle and has been used effectively to limit weight gain in the context of tight control. However, the choice of the pump for insulin delivery requires greater attention to detail and compliance with self-care tasks than any other form of treatment. Therefore, asking the patient to practice the behaviors necessary for success with the insulin pump and assessing the patient's commitment to this expensive and labor-intensive treatment can save resources and prevent unnecessary frustration on the part of the patient and health-care provider. Although the steps listed below are specific to the insulin pump, this approach can be translated to any form of intensified management.

- Evaluate patient motivation and ability regarding the essential tasks associated with pump use using a multiple daily injection routine and self-monitoring of blood glucose.
- Assess patient facility with and psychological comfort regarding use of the pump using a "loaner" pump.
- Assess the patient's intention to use the pump as a long-term method of insulin delivery.
- Assess whether the patient has the financial resources necessary for the maintenance of pump therapy. If finances prevent long-term use

of this treatment method, help the patient identify acceptable therapeutic alternatives.

Assessing Psychological Status

Psychological status can impact a patient's ability to carry out the behavior and the communication necessary to implement and maintain intensive diabetes management. Evaluation of current and prior psychiatric status by a mental health professional who is familiar with diabetes and its care should be included with the assessment of the patient's physical status. Assessment of psychological status should predate intensification, particularly because of the relationship between glucose counterregulation and any form of stress.

- The prior or current diagnosis of a psychiatric illness that impairs an individual's ability to carry out activities of daily living (including diabetes self-care tasks); make, evaluate, or implement treatment decisions; or maintain close contact with a provider is a potential contraindication to intensification.
- If the patient and provider wish to proceed with intensification, appropriate psychosocial supports, including treatment for the psychological issues that may affect treatment and safeguards to monitor treatment efficacy, should be put in place as intensification of care is begun.

Source of motivation for intensive management should also be assessed. If motivation comes from a source outside of the individual, such as the parent of an adolescent or a spouse, the dynamics of that relationship should be assessed because they contribute to the success of treatment. Patients old enough to assume primary responsibility for their diabetes care need to make a commitment to and be supported in the self-care behaviors necessary to achieve good control. Patient commitment to intensive management should be directly assessed by the health-care provider. Unless a commitment is made, diabetes management may become a vehicle for family conflict. Family support is often a critical element in the success of intensive management, because family members provide both concrete resources and emotional support of a patient's effort to improve his or her diabetes care. The process of intensifying treatment should be slowed and the health-care provider should consider referral for counseling if family conflict around diabetes care is manifested.

Although patients with diabetes are not different in their overall rates of psychiatric illness than patients without diabetes, depression is often associated in this population with perceived treatment failure, the burden of the illness, and its treatment. The occurrence of complications that produce functional limitations, such as worsening eyesight or mobility resulting from micro- and macrovascular disease, are also sources of transient depression, lessening of self-esteem and quality of life.

Intensive management in particular places greater burden on the patient than conventional management, creating the potential for "burn out," perceived failure, lowered self-esteem, and consequent depression. Depressive symptoms are associated with both the illness and the treatment.

Another source of unhappines or discontent may be the weight gain that can occur secondary to improved control. Satisfaction with body image, particularly in adolescent and adult women, may diminish, resulting in intentional worsening of control in order to lose weight through calorie wastage via glycosuria. In extreme cases, an eating disorder must be considered when patients manipulate insulin or purge to rid themselves of excess calories while maintaining acceptable glycohemoglobin levels and body weight. Patients who exhibit eating disorders are placing themselves at increased risk when on a tight control regimen, in that manipulation of either calories or insulin or falsification of records to hide elevated blood glucose levels further increases the risk of hypoglycemia and/or diabetic ketoacidosis.

■ Patients should be monitored for signs of depression throughout the course of treatment, because depression will affect motivation and ability to carry out the prescribed regimen. Depression may be manifest in less-frequent self-care behaviors or loss of interest in intensive management.

■ Patients, especially young adult and adolescent women, should be monitored for signs of aberrant eating patterns, manipulation of insulin dose and/or falsification of records when an eating disorder is suspected.

When signs of depression or an eating disorder are apparent, referral to a mental health professional is indicated. Glycemic targets may need to be modified, and appropriate psychosocial supports put in place to ensure the safety of the patient. These supports may include, but are not limited to, antidepressant medications, hospitalization for monitoring of food intake in conjunction with insulin dose, and the initiation of psychotherapy and/or enlisting a family member to monitor the patient's eating habits. If counseling or psychotherapy is initiated, the therapist should be included as part of the diabetes treatment team. They can help monitor the patient's ability to maintain self-care behaviors and assess the patient's psychosocial support system and the impact of the treatment regimen on the patient's mood.

ASSESSING THE EFFECT OF STRESS ON GLYCEMIC CONTROL

It is important to assess the level of stressors—positive and negative—in the patient's life to determine the impact of stress on the individual's ability to maintain good glycemic control. The patient's response to and typical level of stress should be assessed before intensification is begun.

■ Transient stress has the effect of

causing underinsulinization by producing counterregulatory hormones and, consequently, causing hyperglycemia.

- The effects of chronic stress on glycemic control are not well understood. However, repeated sequential stress (physical or psychological) and repeated episodes of hypoglycemia alter counterregulatory response, which may in turn alter the symptoms patients have come to associate with hypoglycemia or anxiety.
- Changed, missing, or blunted counterregulatory response may affect the individual's ability to identify symptoms associated with changes in blood glucose and those due to psychosocial stress.

The identification of stress-related events and symptoms is important in identifying potential causes of high or fluctuating blood glucose levels, especially when tight control is the goal of treatment.

Help patients who strive for tight control to evaluate the effects of stressful life events on blood glucose through the use of careful blood glucose monitoring records in which the patient is encouraged to record life events as well as blood glucose level and insulin dose.

- Assist the patient in learning how to distinguish symptoms caused by life stress (which may in turn affect blood glucose levels) from those that might be expected from primary changes in blood glucose levels (such as feelings of hunger and light-headedness before a planned meal).
- Patients practicing intensive management should be encouraged to test blood glucose whenever they feel symptoms or experience psychosocial stress to identify their own pattern of glycemic response.

Once life events that are stressful and patterns of glycemic response are identified, patient and provider can develop coping strategies that help the patient to maintain acceptable levels of blood glucose.

Although stressful lifestyles do not preclude an intensive diabetes manage-ment regimen, a patient must learn to cope effectively with changes in blood glucose levels caused by stressors and to develop and practice compensatory or substitute behaviors. Intervention strategies for stress reduction can include relaxation techniques, regular exercise regimens, support people/ groups, medications, and changes in the diabetes regimen itself. Intervention strategies should be tailored to the source of the stress, the patient's glycemic response, and the resources (psychological and other) the patient possesses to cope with the stressor.

- With the patient, identify the source(s) of the stress.
- With the patient, quantify the glycemic and emotional response to the stress.
- Suggest and try out coping methods (such as relaxation techniques) that the patient finds acceptable.
- Monitor the effectiveness of the coping strategy and its effect on blood glucose.
- Reevaluate the patient's subjective level of stress and make changes to coping methods as needed to improve glycemic control and emotional well-being.

Patterns of eating in response to stress also need to be addressed, especially in individuals with non-insulin-dependent (type II) diabetes, whose glucose levels can be controlled by caloric intake. Regardless of the type of diabetes, long-term modification of eating habits, including stress-reactive eating, is widely recognized as the most difficult piece of the diabetes-care regimen for the patient to modify. If stress-related eating is identified, the patient will need counseling regarding the skills necessary to maintain glucose levels within the acceptable range through exercise, insulin, or medication modifications. Individualized long-term nutritional and psychological counseling should be offered as an adjunct to short-term strategies aimed at immediate glucose control. The ultimate goal of the intervention should be a lifestyle change, in this case eating or exercise habits, rather than an accommodation to the dysfunctional coping pattern, e.g., adding extra insulin that would result in weight gain. When stress is identified as the cause for overeating, worsening blood glucose level control, or regimen noncompliance, it is appropriate to consider referral to the mental health professional on the health-care team.

ASSESSING COPING SKILLS

Assessment of Diabetes-Related Coping

Effective diabetes-related coping involves

- identifying those factors contributing to current and near-future glycemic status, e.g., life stress, physical stress, calorie intake, exercise, alcohol use, insulin dose, and pump failure
- having the knowledge and skills to evaluate the circumstances and respond appropriately, and
- having access to and willingness to use a health-care professional or support person who can help solve problems and collaborate in a treatment decision.

These coping skills can be taught and practiced. However, assessment of the patient's willingness to take responsibility for treatment decisions or to use a support person to aid in decision making can help avoid adverse events, such as severe hypoglycemia or ketoacidosis due to under- or overtreatment of glucose level. During routine management visits, the patient's willingness to assume responsibility for regimen changes should be reevaluated to prevent "burn out" caused by the intensive diabetes regimen. The patient's ability to cope with life events unrelated to having diabetes should be monitored, along with his or her ability to cope with the requirements of intensive management. Referral to ancillary resources such as support groups and mental health professionals can help foster coping skills and prevent "burn out."

If a pattern of trusting communication has been established between the patient and caregivers, diabetes-related coping strategies can be tried by the patient in the context of the safety net provided by the support system. Once competence is reached in the patient's ability to solve problems related to his or her glucose control, it is the task of the caregiver to shift the responsibility of management decisions to the patient. Increased practice with diabetes-related problem solving and effective self-care behaviors will increase the patient's ability to cope with the effects of stressful life events. Effective self-care behavior will contribute to overall glycemic control and feelings of diabetes-related self-confidence/efficacy and well-being. It is important to note that providers should remain accessible and available for ongoing consultation by the patient regarding management decisions.

Identifying Psychosocial Resources

Interpersonal support, or lack thereof, often determines a patient's ability to implement and maintain intensive management. Psychosocial support often helps remove barriers to adherence as it eases the burden of illness.

- Support can come from a variety of sources: the health-care team, a specific provider, a supportive family member, a religious organization, or a diabetes support group.
- Support can be offered as emotional support that affirms a patients' desire to intensify their diabetes care and to improve their health; as support in treatment decisions; or more concretely, as provision of resources, e.g., financial aid (health-care providers are often able to identify rebate programs from pharmaceutical companies or may put patients in touch with discount supply companies) or physical help with self-care behaviors.

A patient's need for support varies in the same manner that an individual's response to stress varies. Most patients need education about available resources. Management visits can be used to help identify the psychosocial resources in the patient's community. Although patients may be familiar with support groups such as those sponsored by the American Diabetes Association, they may not realize that educational programs and regional support groups are routinely available and that hospitals in the community offer diabetes-care specialty teams.

- Ask patients to identify individuals in their lives who would be willing to be educated to and help with intensive diabetes management.
- Include significant others in the planning of diabetes-care regimens.
- Encourage patients to share the responsibilities of diabetes care with family and friends to whatever extent they feel comfortable.
- Stress that intensive management of diabetes brings the increased risk of severe hypoglycemia, and involving others in diabetes care can provide safeguards against this type of risk.

HELPING PATIENTS DEAL WITH COMPLICATIONS

Much of what patients believe about the inevitability of complications associated with diabetes predates the knowledge that good control can prevent or reduce their occurrence. As shown by the DCCT, serious complications, such as blindness or amputations, are no longer certain outcomes of diabetes. However, many patients continue to hold these beliefs and express feelings of helplessness with regard to altering the course of their illness. If a patient's behavior has not succeeded in achieving good glycemic control, then negative attitudes, such as those regarding a lack of control over complications, may be reinforced. These attitudes should be addressed as part of the intensification process. Successful experience with intensive regimen behaviors, such as

adjustment of insulin dose in response to current glycemia, can change the patient's attitude about the efficacy of the treatment. Success with short-term goals can help alter the patient's attitudes about the inevitability of complications and bolster intentions to continue intensive management.

Complications can exact a psychological toll and may affect a patient's ability to carry out intensive management. Physical limitations or inability to recognize glycemic status secondary to complications should be directly discussed with the patient to develop realistic goals for intensification of diabetes management.

Patients often begin to see themselves as handicapped or limited in their ability to carry out an intensive diabetes-care regimen once complications are diagnosed. Coping with complications that are related to symptom recognition, such as blunted catecholamine response or autonomic neuropathy, may prove difficult for the patient, because they directly affect the patient's ability to assess glycemic level and recognize hypoglycemia. Education regarding different treatment approaches and supports can help renew the patient's commitment to achieving better glycemic control. Patients may need help understanding that any improvement in their glycemic status can improve their health status and help retard the onset and development of further complications.

Complications secondary to intensive management must also be presented to the patient. A good example of this situation is the transient worsening in retinopathy that some patients experience on tightening of glucose control. Although this worsening is transient in many cases, it becomes difficult for the health-care provider to continue to encourage, and for the patient to follow, the same course of action. Patients should be educated to known complications of treatment at the outset of intensification, so that potential worsening of physical status can be anticipated and appropriate emotional and regimen support can be provided during transition periods. Adverse events commonly associated with intensive management are

- worsening retinopathy
- weight gain
- severe hypoglycemia, and
- hypoglycemia unawareness.

These adverse outcomes may result in intentional worsening of control on the part of the patient. Patients need to develop regimen strategies and emotional supports to cope with these possibilities and maintain a long-term perspective. When improved glycemic control is accompanied by hypoglycemia unawareness, or when patients experience a change, a blunting, or a lack of symptoms, increased monitoring of blood glucose should be recommended, and consideration should be given to modifying glycemic targets until hypoglycemia awareness is achieved. Symptom recognition is a critical element in tight control, because the margin of error for recognition of low blood glucose is smaller and the threshold for symptom production also may change with a lower mean level of blood glucose. If hypoglycemia unawareness is secondary to concerted efforts to achieve near-normal glucose levels, patients may need support in accepting modified goals of treatment.

- Teach patients to recognize patterns of hypoglycemia through the use of symptom logs, in conjunction with glucose meters that have a memory function.
- Identify the timing, type, or absence of symptoms in relation to actual glucose levels.
- Help the patient develop compensatory coping strategies, including self-care or lifestyle changes to anticipate periods of expected low blood glucose.

HELPING PATIENTS WITH LONG-TERM ADHERENCE

One of the considerations that has traditionally dissuaded practitioners from intensifying their patients' care regimen is the well-documented and widely held belief that the more complex the treatment regimen, the poorer the compliance. We now know that poor adherence may be the result of a number of factors, in addition to treatment complexity, including

- barriers to adherence, such as lack of resources or accessibility to care
- lack of clarity and poor communication of expected behaviors or regimen prescription
- lack of patient motivation or efficacy, and
- patient nonparticipation in the treatment contract.

Initiation of intensive management of diabetes may be driven by the patient or the provider. However, if patient and provider do not agree on the methods and goals of treatment, if the appropriate education and resources are not provided or available, or if the patient is unable (for whatever functional or practical reason) to carry out the treatment tasks, then treatment "failure" probably will occur. Health-care providers traditionally have attributed treatment failure to "noncompliance" on the part of the patient.

It is necessary to establish a common understanding between the health-care team and the patient of what self-care behaviors, allocation of resources (financial and other), and patterns of communication are expected or required to achieve tight control of blood glucose levels. Patients are often afraid to tell their health-care provider that they feel incapable of carrying out the requested behavior, are disinclined because of fear or lack of resources, or disagree with the regimen prescription in the first place. A patient's willingness to use the education and resources provided by caregivers is crucial to implement intensive management. Patients who do not feel rapport with their caregivers are less likely to incorporate and sustain changes to their care regimen. A patient's willingness to use the resources provided by caregivers also is necessary to help prevent adverse events secondary to the treatment, such as severe hypoglycemia. Establishing an atmosphere of collaboration and mutual respect will help to obtain the patient's cooperation with regard to the intention to carry out the treatment plan, and follow the advice given by the provider.

- Include patients and their support network in the treatment team.
- Define and agree on treatment goals and the self-care behaviors that are expected to achieve and maintain these goals. Monitor and redefine goals as necessary.
- Have patients practice self-care behavior. Provide the necessary education, support, and training for skill acquisition.
- Adapt regimen to lifestyle. Include the patient in regimen choices.
- Make regimen changes incrementally.
- Expect periods of lessened adherence.

Note that treatment behaviors that have been mutually agreed to may not always result in the expected glycemic outcome. Factors such as stress reactivity, other disease processes, or changes in lifestyle or routine may result in regimen effects that are unanticipated. Caregivers and patients engaged in achieving tight control should not view unanticipated outcomes as failures of treatment or noncompliance. Instead, patient and caregiver can work to identify causal relationships between lifestyle, emotion, and glycemic status to develop self-care coping strategies. For example, stress produced by school or job-related responsibilities can cause a rise in blood glucose. The individual may have completed self-care tasks as prescribed and may have attempted to compensate for anticipated stress by extra blood tests or extra insulin/less food. These strategies may not have the anticipated effect on blood glucose, or may produce an effect later in the day. The response can be documented and used as data to decide future treatment plans. It is important to help the patient understand that this should not be viewed as a personal failure, poor problem solving, or treatment failure.

SUPPORTING PATIENTS' BEHAVIOR CHANGES

Mastery of the care behaviors necessary to implement and maintain tight control may be sequential and incremental in an intensive diabetes-care regimen. As each skill is mastered, new skills can be added until the patient achieves the desired glucose goals. An example of this technique is the gradual addition of daily insulin injections into the patient's regimen, along with concurrent blood tests and dosage adjustments. As each additional injection is added to the regimen, the patient's comfort and ability to carry out the behavior are monitored, as is the effectiveness of the new intervention. Practice and success with these behaviors increase the patient's confidence and intentions to continue intensive management, as long as adequate supports are provided. Motivation to initiate intensive management may come from health-care providers, a family member, or the patients themselves. However, patient motivation, ability, and intention to maintain a complex regimen will vary over time. Health-care providers should enlist all possible supports for their patients to lessen the burden of treatment.

- Ongoing education and training in skill acquisition, including diabetes-related problem solving, are necessary components of intensive management.
- Treatment goals should be defined, monitored, and redefined as indicated by patient success with each task.
- Lapses in self-care behaviors should be expected as a routine part of care.

Intensification of diabetes management requires the patient to prioritize the diabetes-care regimen. Ongoing adherence with the diet and exercise portions of the diabetes-care regimen are most difficult for many patients, whether they are using oral medication or insulin or can potentially achieve glycemic control without use of medication. Like other areas targeted for behavior change, diet and exercise require ongoing long-term monitoring and modification of treatment goals according to the patient's success with the intervention strategy.

Helping patients formulate a regimen that is responsive to lifestyle needs will help ensure greater compliance with the prescribed treatment. A treatment regimen that fits into, rather than controls, lifestyle can be constructed. Patients can be instructed on self-care behaviors that respond to current glucose value, activity and exercise, and planned caloric intake.

CONCLUSION

Intensive management offers the patient flexibility of lifestyle and the opportunity to enhance the quality of diabetes-related and general well-being. The importance of psychosocial and medical supports in facilitating the implementation and maintenance of intensive diabetes management should not be underestimated. The availability of multidisciplinary services and support can relieve the patient and the family of some of the burden of diabetes care. Through the incorporation of the patient and the psychosocial support system into the care team, individualized lifestyle-based regimens can be formulated, self-care behaviors can be practiced, and treatment goals can be chosen and monitored. Each patient will require an individualized treatment regimen and a unique constellation of support services, depending on age, social circumstance, psychological status, and financial resources. Some patients are not appropriate candidates for intensive complex treatment regimens. However, diabetes management with the goal of achieving near-normal blood glucose levels can be implemented incrementally, and glycemic targets can be modified based on ongoing monitoring of treatment efficacy. The practice of intensive management of diabetes requires the commitment and dedication of the patient and health-care team on an ongoing long-term basis.

BIBLIOGRAPHY

American Diabetes Association position statement: Standards of medical care for patients with diabetes mellitus. *Diabetes Care* 17:616–23, 1994

Anderson RM: Patient empowerment and the traditional medical model: a case of irreconcilable differences? *Diabetes Care* 18:412–15, 1995

Clarke WL, Gonder-Frederick LA, Richards FE, Cryer PE: Multifactorial origin of hypoglycemic symptom unawareness in IDDM: association with defective glucose counterregulation and better glycemic control. *Diabetes* 40:680–85, 1991

Glasgow RE, Osteen VL: Evaluating diabetes outcomes: are we measuring the most important outcomes? *Diabetes Care* 15: 1423–32, 1992

Greenfield S, Kaplan SH, Ware JE, Yamo EM, Frank H: Patient's participation in medical care: effects on blood sugar control and quality of life in diabetes. *J Gen Intern Med* 3:448–57, 1992

Jacobson AM: Depression and diabetes. *Diabetes Care* 16:1621–23, 1993

Lustman PJ, Frank BL, McGill JB: Relationship of personality characteristics to glucose regulation in adults with diabetes. *Psychosom Med* 53:305–12, 1991

Mazze RS, Eztwiler DD, Strock E, Peterson K, McClare CR II, Meszzros JF, Leigh C, Owens LW, Deeb LC, Peterson A, Kummer M: Staged diabetes management: toward an integrated model of diabetes care. *Diabetes Care* 17 (Suppl. 1):56–66, 1994

McCulloch DK, Glasgow RE, Hampson SE, Wagner E: A systematic approach to diabetes management in the post-DCCT era. *Diabetes Care* 17:765–69, 1994

Rodin GM, Daneman D: Eating disorders and IDDM: a problematic association. *Diabetes Care* 15: 1402–12, 1992

Schafer LC, Glasgow RE, McCaul

KD, Dreher M: Adherence to IDDM regimens: relationship to psychosocial variables and metabolic control. *Diabetes Care* 6:493–98, 1983

Spilker B, Cramer JA (Eds.): *Patient Compliance in Medical Practice and Clinical Trials.* New York, Raven, 1991

Surwit RS, Schneider MS, Feinglos MN: Stress and diabetes mellitus. 15:1413–22, 1992

Patient Selection and Goals of Therapy

Highlights

Patient Selection
Patients With Type I Diabetes
Patients With Type II Diabetes

Goals of Therapy
Glycemic Goals
Modifying Glycemic Goals
Weighing Benefits and Risks In Type II Diabetes

Highlights
Patient Selection and
Goals of Therapy

■ Appropriate patient selection is crucial to the success and safety of any treatment regimen. A successful intensive diabetes management program must be a diabetes self-management program.

■ Patient characteristics that influence success of intensive diabetes management are
  ■ willingness to be actively involved in care
  ■ desire to improve glycemic control
  ■ access to adequate diabetes education
  ■ acceptable balance between treatment-associated risks and benefits
  ■ ongoing communication with health-care team, and
  ■ presence of adequate support networks.

■ A successful treatment regimen is adaptable to meet lifestyle needs, balances the patient's risks and benefits, and is subject to ongoing evaluation and modification.

■ No one set of glycemic goals can be applied to every person with diabetes. Glycemic targets must be modified according to the patient's age, disease duration, type of diabetes, prior hypoglycemia history, lifestyle/occupation, diabetes complications status, concurrent medical conditions, and support network.

■ If intensive diabetes management is deemed unacceptable or inadvisable for a particular patient, efforts must still be made to encourage whatever degree of glycemic improvement is individually and safely possible.

Patient Selection and Goals of Therapy

A successful intensive diabetes management program must be a diabetes self-management program. The relative effectiveness of intensive management efforts is influenced by certain patient characteristics.

PATIENT SELECTION

Appropriate patient selection is crucial to the success and safety of any treatment regimen. However, the guidelines for patient selection cannot be rigidly defined. Instead, assessment of suitability for intensive diabetes management needs to be individualized, based on objective and subjective information provided by both the patient and the health-care team (Table 5.1).

Patients need to feel that they have options and that they are involved in the decisions that affect their health care. The health belief model offers some useful insights to consider when dealing with individuals who have diabetes (Table 5.2).

Not all individuals with diabetes will be equally motivated to become more actively involved in their management. For some patients, injecting insulin once or twice a day or taking a couple pills will be the maximum extent of their desired involvement. For these patients, it is crucial to determine whether their decision is an informed one, based on adequate access to objective information. Once receipt of this information is confirmed, the continued decision to remain detached from self-care must be acknowledged and accepted by the health-care team, ensuring that the patient is neither neglected nor made to feel guilty for the decision. Motivation to improve self-care cannot be forced. Ultimately, the control of diabetes resides with the individual who has diabetes. However, health-care providers are encouraged to acknowledge whatever positive changes are made and to continue to evaluate the patient for readiness to make more significant changes as time progresses.

An individual's ability to make reasonable and informed decisions is influenced by knowledge of the pros and cons associated with each decision. Before committing to intensive diabetes management, the patient must be adequately informed of the risks, as well as the benefits, associated with intensive therapy in a balanced manner. Decisions about the appropriateness of individual patients for intensive diabetes management and discussions of the potential benefits and risks should be

---

Table 5.1. Patient Characteristics That Influence the Success of Intensive Diabetes Management Efforts

- Competency and involvement in current self-care program
- Willingness to become *actively* involved in daily management
- Desire to improve glycemic control
- Educated regarding diabetes self-management techniques
- Acceptance of benefits and risks associated with intensive management
- Willingness to engage in ongoing open and honest communication with health-care team
- Recognition of physical and emotional abilities; able to effectively communicate with health-care team and carry out treatment tasks
- Presence of personal and health-care support networks

Table 5.2. Health Belief Model

People are more likely to follow treatment recommendations if

- They feel that they are vulnerable to the disease and/or its consequences
- They feel that the disease could have a negative effect on their life
- They feel that following the treatment recommendations will reduce their risks
- They feel that the benefits of the treatment outweigh its risks and/or costs

undertaken by a health-care team that is not only knowledgeable about the pertinent literature related to intensive management but also experienced in its implementation. The health-care provider must present an honest review of perceived benefits and risks and should not be judgmental or critical of the patient's decision to implement or not to implement intensive diabetes management.

Once the commitment to improved glycemic control using intensive diabetes management has been made, the patient must have access to education regarding diabetes self-management techniques (see DIABETES SELF-MANAGEMENT EDUCATION).

In addition, the patient must be physically and emotionally capable of meeting the more rigorous demands of the intensive diabetes management regimen. Health-care providers need to be sensitive to the fact that not all individuals will meet these demands in the same way. The patient's age and the family's support, as well as the intellectual, emotional, financial, occupational, and domestic status of a patient, need to be taken into account when customizing an intensive treatment regimen and choosing glycemic targets.

- Does the patient have the financial resources to pay for the costs associated with intensive treatment, e.g., doctor and hospital visits, transportation, testing, equipment, and supplies?
- Is the patient self-sufficient or mature enough to assume primary responsibility for care and treatment decisions?
- If the patient is not, is there a responsible individual who is willing to be educated and to actively participate in a more complex time-consuming care regimen?
- If the patient lives alone, who will have daily or frequent contact with the patient in case of emergencies, such as severe hypoglycemia or illness requiring outside intervention?
- Does the patient's domestic and work/study environment permit and support the behaviors necessary to carry out intensive treatment?

Ongoing assessment of the patient's ability to achieve defined treatment goals and integrate the regimen into daily life should guide decisions to alter the regimen. If any issues impair the patient's ability to carry out or monitor the effects of treatment, then regimen tasks, prescription, and/or glycemic targets should be modified.

A motivated patient and knowledgeable health-care team collaborate in creating a management plan with individually defined treatment methods and goals. The regimen must be adaptable to meet the individual's lifestyle needs, must carefully balance the risks and benefits of therapy, and must be subjected to ongoing evaluation and modification. To ensure accurate and current evaluation, the patient must be willing to commit to maintaining regular contact with the health-care team. Through this frequent contact, effective changes can be made and problem-solving skills can be developed.

For many patients, intensive management efforts enhance lifestyle flexibility and promote a sense of control over diabetes. However, tight control of blood glucose levels can be accomplished by many methods. Therefore, although modifications to an intensive treatment regimen may be necessary because of the patient's situation or for psychosocial reasons, glycemic control need not be sacrificed.

Patients With Type I Diabetes

Intensive diabetes management should be considered for most individuals with type I diabetes. Implementation is strongly recommended for particular individuals

- motivated individuals, with or without early evidence of complications, and
- women who are pregnant or are contemplating pregnancy.

Caution and care should be exercised when determining whether to pursue intensive treatment for specific subsets of the type I population (Table 5.3). All treatment decisions must weigh the benefits of the treatment against the associated risks, with the resulting balance dictating the treatment strategies and goals. When assessment indicates unsuitability for implementation of intensive therapy, then efforts still should be made to encourage whatever degree of glycemic improvement is possible.

Patients With Type II Diabetes

Intensive diabetes management also should be considered for individuals with type II diabetes. Although the pharmacological treatment modalities may differ from those for individuals with type I diabetes, frequent blood glucose monitoring, nutrition management, exercise guidelines, and ongoing communication with the health-care team for assessment, education, care, and support remain crucial components of the treatment regimen.

Current treatment strategies employed in the care of individuals with type II diabetes require scrutiny. If patients are to accept the seriousness of their condition, then their health-care providers must review their management approach to type II diabetes and be cognizant of the message that patients receive when told, "You only have a touch of sugar," "Just follow your diet, and/or lose a bit of weight, and everything will be fine," or "You just have borderline diabetes."

The myth that type II diabetes is a less serious, less debilitating disease than type I diabetes, because daily injections are not needed to sustain life, continues to influence treatment decisions. Several points must be made in this regard.

- Epidemiological data implicate hyperglycemia as a risk factor for macrovascular disease.
- Macrovascular disease is responsible for major morbidity and mortality in individuals with type II diabetes.
- Nearly 40% of individuals with type II diabetes are treated with insulin.

Table 5.3. Patient Characteristics That Negatively Influence Risk-Benefit Ratio in Intensive Type I Diabetes Management

- Individuals with hypoglycemia unawareness
- Individuals with a history of recurrent severe hypoglycemic episodes
- Individuals with impaired counterregulatory response to hypoglycemia
- Individuals requiring medications that may interfere with hypoglycemia detection and/or treatment, i.e., ß-blockers
- Individuals with severe emotional disorders or psychosocial stressors
- Individuals with alcohol- or drug-abuse problems
- Individuals with advanced, end-stage diabetic complications
- Individuals with other medical conditions that can be aggravated by hypoglycemia, i.e., cerebrovascular disease or angina
- Children under the age of 10
- Individuals unable or unwilling to commit to the personal effort and involvement required for intensive diabetes management

---

The patient characteristics listed in Table 5.1 also should be considered when assessing the appropriateness of patients with type II diabetes for intensive management implementation. Special consideration should be given to individuals included in the categories listed in Table 5.4. These issues represent relative considerations, not absolute contraindications, for intensive therapy implementation. Again, if the patient is not an appropriate candidate for intensive management, efforts still should be made to improve

---

Table 5.4. Patient Characteristics That Negatively Influence Risk-Benefit Ratio in Intensive Type II Diabetes Management

- Individuals with symptomatic coronary artery disease
- Individuals with cardiac arrhythmias
- Individuals with concurrent diseases and/or conditions that would functionally limit intensive management, i.e., debilitating arthritis or severe visual impairment
- Individuals with relatively short life expectancy

Table 5.5. Goals of Therapy for All People With Diabetes, Independent of Blood Glucose Targets

- Avoid life-threatening acute metabolic imbalance, including
  - Diabetic ketoacidosis
  - Hyperosmolar hyperglycemic nonketotic coma
  - Dehydration
  - Severe hypoglycemia
- Prevent hospitalization
- Minimize symptoms related to hyperglycemia
- Minimize symptomatic hypoglycemia that disrupts activities
- Achieve normal linear growth and sexual development (for children)
- Maintain appropriate body weight (for all patients)
- Accomplish normal school attendance, job performance, or social activities

Table 5.6. Factors to Consider in Establishing Individualized Treatment Goals

- Age
- Disease duration
- Type of diabetes (type I, type II, or gestational)
- Prior hypoglycemia history
  - History of severe hypoglycemia
  - Ability to recognize hypoglycemic symptoms
- Lifestyle and occupation, e.g., What are the consequences of experiencing hypoglycemia on the job?
- Are complications of diabetes already present, and how severe are they?
- Are there other medical conditions or treatments present that might alter the response to therapy?
- What level of support from family and friends is available?

GOALS OF THERAPY

Before approaching the specific glycemic targets of intensive diabetes management, it is important to emphasize some general goals of diabetes therapy, other than those that are directly related to blood glucose level (Table 5.5).

It would be meaningless to set primarily blood glucose targets for the patient who is incapacitated by diabetes to the point of being unable to work or attend school because of recurrent diabetic ketoacidosis and/or severe hypoglycemia (termed *brittle diabetes*). For such patients, establishing a healthy, safe, and productive lifestyle should be primary and specific glycemic targets sought only after these more basic goals have been accomplished. Although some of these patients may respond favorably to intensive diabetes management, this is not universally the case. Most patients classified as brittle have poor compliance and/or psychological or psychiatric problems as a significant, if not primary, cause of their instability. Likewise, it would be inappropriate to set glycemic targets that could be accomplished only by interference with normal day-to-day life (e.g., preventing normal attendance at school or on the job) either because of too many restrictions or because of too-frequent symptomatic hypoglycemia.

No single set of goals or target blood glucose levels can be applied to every person with diabetes. What might be recommended for an otherwise healthy young adult with type I diabetes early in the course of the illness may differ markedly from what is recommended for an older adult with coronary artery disease and reduced vision or for a toddler with working parents who spends most of the day in a day-care setting. Factors that play a role in determining the goals for any patient include age, duration of diabetes, type of diabetes, prior history of hypoglycemia, lifestyle or occupation, presence or absence of complications, other medical conditions or treatments, and availability of support from family or friends (Table 5.6).

glycemic control as much as is safely possible. Treatment decisions and goals also must incorporate the presence and management requirements of associated risk factors for macrovascular disease, such as hypertension, hypercholesterolemia, or weight gain.

Glycemic Goals

Glycemic targets for intensive diabetes management are presented in Table 5.7. These goals, supported by the American Diabetes Association, are less ambitious than those selected for the intensively treated patients in the Diabetes Control and Complications Trial (DCCT). In the DCCT, despite the best efforts of carefully selected patients and highly motivated staff, the glycemic targets were accomplished consistently by only a few patients.

Not incorporated into these recommended goals is the need to determine overnight blood glucose levels to assess the presence of nocturnal hypoglycemia. Most of the severe hypoglycemic episodes in the DCCT occurred overnight (43%) or during sleep (55%). A lower limit for overnight blood glucose should be added to these goals. The frequently used value is 65 mg/dl (3.6 mM). However, if the patient is known to experience severe hypoglycemia symptoms or impaired cognitive function at blood glucose levels in the 60s, then the acceptable nocturnal level should be higher.

For many teenage and young adult patients with type I diabetes who are otherwise healthy, some episodes of mild hypoglycemia usually are considered acceptable, as long as they are well recognized and appropriately treated before severe hypoglycemia occurs and are not so frequent as to interfere with day-to-day life. Even mild hypoglycemia needs to be avoided during operation of a motor vehicle or complex machinery and in those with a reduced counterregulatory response to hypoglycemia (defective glucose counterregulation) or hypoglycemia unawareness. These conditions may come about secondary to recurrent episodes of mild hypoglycemia in some patients (hypoglycemia-associated autonomic failure); these patients need to avoid even mild hypoglycemia.

Modifying Glycemic Goals

Glycemic targets must be individualized. Specific situations requiring goals other than those noted in Table 5.7 are summarized in Table 5.8. For example, adults whose occupation requires continual mental alertness and quick reaction time for purposes of their safety or the safety of others need to be especially cautious to avoid hypoglycemia and may need to raise the glycemic goals somewhat. In addition, even in the absence of these specific situations, glycemic goals should be modified based on the level of understanding and motivation of the patient and the support network of family and friends.

Pregnancy
During pregnancy, a lower glycemic target range is often recommended.

Table 5.7. Glycemic Control for People With Diabetes

BIOCHEMICAL INDEX	NONDIABETIC	GOAL	ACTION SUGGESTED
Preprandial glucose (mg/dl)	<115 (<6.4 mM)	80-120 (4.4-6.7 mM)	<80 (<4.4 mM) or >140 (>7.8 mM)
Bedtime glucose (mg/dl)	<120 (<6.7 mM)	100-140 (5.6-7.8 mM)	<100 (<5.6 mM) or >160 (>8.9 mM)
HbA_{1c} (%)*	<6	<7	>8

*Results vary depending on assay method used.

Many endocrinologists or obstetricians who treat high-risk patients may suggest preprandial glucose levels of 70–100 mg/dl (3.9–5.6 mM) and postprandial glucose levels <140 mg/dl (<7.8 mM), with the mean glucose level over the day being 70–100 mg/dl (3.9–5.6 mM). Accomplishment of these targets requires even more effort on the part of the patient and the health-care team than that of intensive therapy in other settings. Avoidance of hypoglycemia must still be considered an important goal.

Children
The prior history of severe hypoglycemia and the potential danger for permanent sequelae associated with severe hypoglycemia need to be considered carefully when setting individualized glycemic targets. The best example of this occurs in very young children, usually under 6–7 yr of age. For young children, with a developing CNS, significant hypoglycemia may be associated with a minor, or perhaps even major, loss of cognitive function that may be permanent. Therefore, the avoidance of hypoglycemia becomes a more important goal in this age-group, and glycemic targets generally are higher. The goal of preprandial glucose levels between 100 and 140 mg/dl (5.6–7.8 mM) would seem more appropriate for children. Once again, however, it is important to individualize the goals.

Table 5.8. Patients Who Require Alterations of Glycemic Goals

- Pregnant women and those planning pregnancy
- Patients with occupations in which the occurrence of hypoglycemia may endanger themselves and others
- Children <7 yr old, in whom the danger of hypoglycemia is increased
- Elderly patients, especially those living alone and those with cardiovascular disease
- Patients with a history of recurrent severe hypoglycemia or hypoglycemia unawareness

Elderly Patients
Goals for therapy in elderly patients warrant special consideration. Many have other complicating therapies or medical conditions, such as cardiovascular disease. Some are visually impaired. Some live alone and have minimal support. The benefits of lowering blood glucose have not been studied in this population and may not be evident during the patient's lifetime. In addition to a less clear definition of benefits in the elderly, the risks (especially those associated with hypoglycemia) may be greater.

Weighing Benefits and Risks in Type II Diabetes

The goals of therapy for patients with type II diabetes also need to be developed with the understanding that the risks and benefits of intensive management in this group are unknown. Some degree of lowering of the blood glucose toward the normal range is desirable. If this can be accomplished by regimens involving diet and nutritional counseling, exercise, oral hypoglycemic agents, and/or simple insulin regimens (e.g., NPH insulin once a day), then a regimen using multiple daily insulin injections may not add benefit. For those requiring the use of more aggressive, or perhaps even intensive, regimens of insulin administration, the glycemic goals of therapy may be similar to those for younger type I patients. However, goals may need to be modified, because of hypoglycemia and/or additional weight gain. Many patients with type II diabetes are already obese, which may contribute to their diabetic state and hyperglycemia as well as their long-term outcome. For some, the risk of additional weight gain or hypoglycemia may outweigh the potential benefits of lowering blood glucose levels.

CONCLUSION

Successful integration of the diabetes regimen requires the melding of the patient's medical management requirements with a willingness and an ability to perform the necessary treatment tasks. Intensified diabetes management efforts should be considered for all individuals with diabetes. However, special consideration is needed for patients whose safety and/or well-being can be compromised if the only goal is perfect glycemic control.

Improved glycemic control for all individuals with diabetes is the desired outcome of treatment interventions. The relationship of glycemic control and long-term complications must be considered in the context of the risks and costs associated with this treatment. However, if treatment strategies are to be effective in reducing long-term sequelae, then treatment goals and implementation techniques must be individualized. Although not all patients will be able to meet the demands of intensive diabetes management, all patients will benefit from any achievable improvement in glycemic control. This should signal the need for ongoing evaluation and encouragement for any degree of improvement or increase in self-care efforts, rather than cause health-care providers to retreat.

No patient should arbitrarily be dismissed as ineligible or unacceptable for intensified management efforts. Instead, each patient should be critically evaluated for the ability and willingness to employ intensive diabetes management, given the requisite knowledge, skills, and resources. In addition, if intensive diabetes management is reasonable for a given patient, but financial constraints prohibit implementation in the current health-care setting, efforts should be made to refer the patient to community resources that may be available to assist the patient in achieving maximally safe and effective glycemic control.

BIBLIOGRAPHY

American Diabetes Association: *Medical Management of Insulin-Dependent Type I Diabetes*. 2nd ed. Santiago JV, Ed. Alexandria, VA, Am. Diabetes Assoc., 1994, p. 16–57

American Diabetes Association: *Therapy for Diabetes Mellitus and Related Disorders*. 2nd ed. Lebonitz HE, Ed. Alexandria, VA, Am. Diabetes Assoc., 1994, p. 131–46

Becker MH, Janz NK: The health belief model applied to understanding diabetics' regimen compliance. *Diabetes Educator* 11: 41–47, 1985

Farkas-Hirsch R: Clinical management of insulin pump therapy. *Pract Diabetol* 11:24–27, 1992

Farkas-Hirsch R, Levandoski L: Implementation of continuous subcutaneous insulin infusion therapy: an overview. *Diabetes Educator* 14:401–406, 1988

Genuth S: Insulin use in NIDDM. *Diabetes Care* 13:1240 64, 1990

Gerich JE: Selection of patients for intensive insulin therapy. *Arch Intern Med* 145:1383–84, 1985

Haakens K, Hanssen KF, Dahl-Jorgensen K, Vaaler S, Aagenaes O, Mosand R: Continuous subcutaneous insulin infusion (CSII), multiple injections (MI) and conventional insulin therapy (CT) in self-selecting insulin-dependent diabetic patients: a comparison of metabolic control, acute complications and patient preferences. *J Intern Med* 228:457–64, 1990

Hirsch IB, Farkas-Hirsch R, Skyler JS: Intensive insulin therapy for treatment of type I diabetes mellitus. *Diabetes Care* 13:1265–83, 1990

Jornsay DL, Duckles AE, Hankinson JP: Psychological considerations for patient selection and adjustment to insulin pump therapy. *Diabetes Educator* 14:291–96, 1988

Marcus AO: Selecting patients for insulin pump therapy. *Pract Diabetol* 11:12–18, 1992

Rosenstock J, Strowig S, Raskin P: Insulin pump therapy: a realistic appraisal. *Clin Diabetes* 3:26-31, 1985

Schade DS, Santiago JV, Skyler JS, Rizza RA: Selection and management of the patient receiving inten- sive insulin therapy. In *Intensive Insulin Therapy*. Princcton, NJ, Excerpta Med.,1983, p.194-208

Skyler JS: Intensive insulin therapy: a personal and historical perspec- tive. *Diabetes Educator* 15:33-39, 1989

Zimmerman BR: Practical aspects of intensive insulin therapy. *Mayo Clin Proc* 61:806-12, 1986

Multiple-Component Insulin Regimens

Highlights

Insulin Pharmacology

Insulin Timing and Action
Stability and Miscibility of Insulins
Insulin Absorption

Insulin Regimens

Multiple-Component Insulin Regimens: General Points
Specific Flexible Multiple-Component Insulin Regimens
Other Intensive (But Less Flexible) Insulin Programs

Insulin Dose and Distribution

Initial Insulin Doses
Insulin Dose Distribution

Insulin Algorithms

Preprandial Algorithms
Pattern-Adjustment Algorithms

Injection Devices

Highlights Multiple-Component Insulin Regimens

- Multiple-component insulin regimens use three types of insulin.
    - Regular insulin has the most rapid onset of action, peak effect, and shortest duration.
    - Intermediate-acting insulin, NPH, and lente have a more delayed onset of action, peak effect, and a longer duration of action.
    - Long-acting insulin (ultra-lente) has the longest action profile.

- Insulin absorption and availability is influenced by several factors
    - anatomical regions of injections, with the fastest absorption from the abdomen and the slowest from the thigh
    - timing of premeal injections, and
    - other factors such as exercise and ambient temperature.

- Use of multiple-component insulin regimens attempts to mimic physiologic insulin release.
    - These consist of various confirmations of basal and prandial insulin components.
    - Frequent self-monitoring of blood glucose (SMBG) levels ensures appropriate changes in insulin dosage and timing, food intake, and activity profile.
    - Preprandial regular insulin is administered by syringe, pen, or insulin pump.
    - Basal insulin is administered by insulin pump or as NPH, lente, or ultralente.

- Specific insulin regimens allow individual, flexible combinations of insulins that are suitable for various lifestyles
    - premeal regular and basal NPH or lente
    - premeal regular and basal ultralente, or
    - continuous subcutaneous insulin infusion.

- Other intensive insulin programs offer less flexibility
    - twice-daily mixtures of regular and NPH or lente or
    - prebreakfast regular and NPH or lente, predinner regular and bedtime NPH or lente.

- Calculation of initial insulin dosages usually range from 0.5 to $1.0 \text{ U} \cdot \text{kg}^{-1}$ body wt $\cdot$ day^{-1}. Dosage requirements can vary considerably during the honeymoon phase, intercurrent illness, adolescence, and pregnancy.

- Insulin dosage is then divided into basal and preprandial injections
    - 40–50% provides basal insulinemia.
    - Remainder is divided among the meals either empirically, by use of counting carbohydrate ratios, or by preset guidelines.
    - All regimens must be individualized to patient's desires, lifestyle, and level of glycemic control needed.

- Insulin algorithms consist of an action plan for the alteration of therapy to achieve individually defined glycemic goals.
    - Changes are made in insulin dosage, timing of injections, or in the meal plan and are guided by SMBG results.
    - Preprandial algorithms consist of anticipatory, given prospectively, or compensatory, given retrospectively, supplements.
    - Pattern-adjustment algorithms consist of modification in the usual or basic insulin dosage in response to a pattern of glycemia.

Multiple-Component Insulin Regimens

This chapter discusses the design and use of insulin regimens for intensive diabetes management.

INSULIN PHARMACOLOGY

Insulin Timing and Action

There are three general categories of time course of insulin action: rapid onset, e.g., regular (soluble) insulin; intermediate acting, e.g., NPH (isophane) or lente (insulin-zinc suspension); and long acting, e.g., ultralente (extended insulin-zinc suspension). Table 6.1 summarizes the nominal time action profiles—time to peak action and duration of action—of these insulin preparations. The values shown are for human insulin. Human insulin has both reduced immunogenicity (i.e., induction of insulin antibodies) and reduced antigenicity (i.e., lower titer of anti-insulin antibodies) compared to animal insulins. Therefore, human insulin has a more predictable time course than ani-mal insulins. There is no obvious circumstance in which human insulin is contraindicated.

A general pharmacokinetic principle is that with longer time to peak, there is a resulting broader peak and longer duration of action. Another principle is that the breadth of the peak and the duration of action will be lengthened somewhat with increasing dose. The values included in Table 6.1 are for doses of 10–15 U, or 0.1–0.2 U/kg.

Regular Insulin
Regular (soluble or unmodified) insulin has the most rapid onset and shortest duration of action of any native insulin preparation. (Note, however, that some insulin analogs, e.g., lys-pro insulin, have been designed to have a more rapid onset and shorter duration of action than regular insulin.) Regular insulin has an onset of action of 15–60 min, a peak effect that occurs 2–4 h after administration, and a duration of action of 4–6 h. Duration of action may be longer when large doses are used or when patients have insulin antibodies.

Table 6.1. Time Course (h) of Action of Insulin Preparation After Subcutaneous Injection

	ONSET	PEAK	DURATION
■ Rapid onset			
Regular (crystalline; soluble)	0–1	2–4	4–6
■ Intermediate acting			
NPH (isophane)	1–4	8–10	12–20
Lente (insulin-zinc suspension)	2–4	8–12	12–20
■ Long acting ultralente	3–5	10–16	18–24
(extended insulin-zinc suspension)			
■ Combinations			
70/30 (70% NPH, 30% regular)	0–1	Dual	12–20
50/50 (50% NPH, 50% regular)	0–1	Dual	12–20

Based on doses of 0.1–0.2 U/kg, in the abdomen, for human insulin.

Intermediate-Acting Insulins

NPH insulin. Neutral Protamine Hagedorn (NPH) insulin, also called isophane insulin, uses protamine to extend insulin action. NPH insulin has an onset of action 1–4 h after administration, a peak effect that occurs 8–10 h after administration, and a duration of action of 12–20 h.

Lente insulin. Lente insulin uses zinc to extend insulin action. The time course of action of lente insulin is similar to NPH insulin, i.e., onset in 2–4 h, peak in 8–12 h, and duration of 12–20 h.

Long–Acting Insulin

Ultralente insulin has the longest action profile. Human (Ultralente) insulin has an onset of action of 3–5 h after administration, a peak effect that occurs in 10–16 h, and a duration of action of 18–24 h.

Insulin Mixtures

There also are preparations of mixtures of regular and NPH insulins. These mixtures contain either 70% NPH and 30% regular insulin (called "70/30") or 50% NPH and 50% regular insulin (called "50/50"). These premixed insulins are helpful in infants and in elderly patients, blind patients, or others who may have difficulty mixing insulin in the syringe. However, because these mixtures limit flexibility, they are not useful for most patients using flexible or intensive insulin programs.

Stability and Miscibility of Insulins

Insulin is stable for long periods if refrigerated. It is best stored in the refrigerator. However, insulin is generally stable at room temperature for 1 mo and does not need to be stored in the refrigerator after the bottle is opened, as long as it is used within 1 mo. On the other hand, it should not be exposed to extremes of temperature, such as might occur if left in a car, near a window, or by a heating or air conditioning vent. It should not be exposed to direct sunlight or heat (including temperatures $>30°C$ [$>86°F$]). Also, insulin should not be frozen.

Only regular insulin is in solution. Other insulin preparations are in suspension. Vials containing insulin suspensions must be gently rolled to assure uniform suspension before insulin is withdrawn from the vial.

Mixtures of two types of insulin vary in stability. Regular and NPH insulins are freely miscible in all proportions. These insulins may be mixed in the same syringe, and their action profiles maintained. Mixtures of regular insulin and either lente or ultralente are not stable in vitro. When regular insulin is mixed with lente or ultralente insulin, the rapidity of onset of action of the regular insulin is blunted, even if the insulin remains in the syringe for as few as 2–10 min. However, most or all of the rapid action is retained if mixing is done in a syringe immediately before injection. Full action is retained if separate syringes are used to inject the insulin through a single needle. Loss of soluble material from such mixtures increases over time (at least up to 24 h) and with increased proportions of lente in the mixture.

For reproducibility and to assure equivalent dosing, it is important to follow routinely from day to day the same technique for measuring insulin dosage, mixing insulins, and administering insulin. If a patient is having significant glycemic excursions surrounding meals and needs more rapid insulin effect, consider that there may be some loss of regular insulin activity. This can be tested by temporarily switching to separate injections. For patients who have their insulin premixed in the syringe by health personnel or family and saved for ≥1 day before use, it is desirable to be sure that an exception is not made on the day that the mixing is actually done. Namely, a visiting nurse premixing insulin for a week should mix the insulin for the day he or she will next visit, so that all syringes have been stored for at least 24 h before use.

Insulin Absorption

Many factors may influence insulin absorption and alter insulin availability. Intraindividual variation in insulin absorption from day to day is ~25%, and between patients, it is up to 50%. Although this variation is approximately the same (in percentage terms) for all insulin preparations, in absolute terms (minutes or hours) there is much less variation in absorption of rapidly absorbed regular insulin and greater variation in absorption of longer-acting insulins. Therefore, insulin regimens that emphasize regular insulin are more reproducible in their effects on blood glucose.

Injection Site
There are regional differences in insulin absorption, especially for rapidly absorbed regular insulin. Absorption is fastest from the abdomen, followed by the arm, buttocks, and thigh. These differences are the likely result of variation in blood flow. The variation is sufficiently great that random rotation of injection sites should be avoided. There should be rotation of injection sites *within* regions, rather than *between* regions for any given injection (e.g., prebreakfast) to decrease day-to-day variability. Because the abdomen has the most rapid insulin absorption (in the absence of exercise), it may be preferred for preprandial injections. Some patients use the abdomen for all preprandial injections, whereas others use the abdomen for prebreakfast injection and other regions for prelunch or presupper injections.

Injection site choice can influence the time course of any given insulin formulation. Choice of injection sites depends on the insulin program and the patient's lifestyle. Thus, if an intermediate-acting insulin is used to provide basal insulin for a long period of the day (≥ 15 h), it is desirable to inject into a site from which absorption is slow, e.g., the thigh. On the other hand, if the intermediate-acting insulin is used to provide basal insulin for a shorter period of the day (e.g., 8–10 h), any injection site may be used. Moreover, if empirically the duration of action of any insulin preparation is longer or shorter than desired, a site may be chosen with faster or slower absorption.

Timing of Premeal Injections
Timing of preprandial insulin injections is crucial to matching insulinemia with glycemic excursions after meals.
- With regular insulin, the injection time optimally is 30–60 min before eating, with 20–30 min being practical. The timing of injections should be altered depending on the level of premeal glycemia.
- When blood glucose levels are above a patient's target range, it may be desirable to increase the interval between insulin administration and meal consumption to permit the insulin to begin to have its effect.
- If premeal blood glucose levels are below a patient's target range, it is desirable to delay the administration of insulin until immediately before meal consumption.

Factors Influencing Insulin Absorption
Physical exercise increases blood flow to an exercising body part and thus accelerates absorption of insulin from that region. Sporadic exercise may induce variability in insulin absorption. The patient should try to avoid injections in a region that will be exercised while that injection is being absorbed. For example, when planning jogging shortly after an injection, the patient should avoid giving that injection into the thigh. When exercise is contemplated, the patient might use the abdomen preferentially, because this is the least likely region to have significant increases in absorption (unless sit-ups are planned).

Other factors influencing absorption of regular insulin are ambient temperature (e.g., a hot bath or sauna), smoking, and local massage of the injection site.

In thin patients, with little subcutaneous tissue, there may be more rapid absorption of any given insulin preparation, because it may be injected intramuscularly rather than subcutaneously. This may result in the need for a different insulin formulation, e.g., human ultralente insulin being used as an intermediate-acting insulin in such patients. Also, the interval between injection of preprandial regular insulin and meal consumption may need to be shortened.

INSULIN REGIMENS

Multiple-Component Insulin Regimens: General Points

Physiologic insulin secretion is of two types: continuous basal insulin secretion and incremental prandial insulin secretion, controlling meal-related glucose excursions (Fig. 6.1). Basal insulin secretion restrains hepatic glucose production, keeping it in equilibrium with basal glucose use by brain and other tissues that are obligate glucose consumers. After meals, prandial insulin secretion stimulates glucose use and storage while inhibiting hepatic glucose output. Patients with type I diabetes lack both basal and prandial insulin secretion. Thus, insulin programs for type I diabetes should have multiple components that attempt to mimic these two normal types of endogenous physiologic insulin secretion, by providing components that

give prandial insulin coinciding with each meal and separate components that provide basal insulinemia overnight and between meals. The most flexible regimens used for intensive diabetes management

- emphasize the need for preprandial insulin before each meal, separate from basal insulin
- allow liberal food choices in terms of size, timing, and potential omission of meals while still balancing food intake with activity and insulin dosage, and
- include frequent monitoring of therapy to promote a more normal lifestyle.

Instrumental to the overall plan is self-monitoring of blood glucose (SMBG) several times daily. The patient takes action on the basis of the SMBG results, which are used to help make appropriate changes in insulin dosage and timing, food intake, and activity profile. The changes are made according to a predetermined plan—a set of algorithms—provided by the health-care team to the patient.

Prandial Insulin Therapy

Prandial incremental insulin secretion is best duplicated by giving preprandial injections of rapid-onset regular insulin before each meal by syringe, pen, or pump. Each preprandial insulin dose is adjusted individually to provide meal insulinemia appropriate to the size of the meal. Thus, the size of the premeal insulin dose parallels the size of the meal. The timing of meals need not be fixed, and meals may be omitted along with the accompanying preprandial insulin dose, which increases flexibility in meal timing.

Regular insulin administered subcutaneously is relatively rapid in its onset of action but not immediate. Therefore, as noted above, it is best to give prandial injections at least 20–30 min (or longer) before eating a given meal in an attempt to have prandial insulinemia parallel meal-related glycemic excursions. (In the future, with the availability of rapid-onset insulin analogs, e.g., lys-pro insulin, it will be possible to inject these at the time of meal consumption.)

Fig. 6.1. Twenty-Four-Hour Plasma Glucose and Insulin Profiles in a Hypothetical Nondiabetic Individual

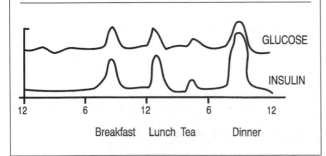

Basal Insulin Therapy

Basal insulinemia is given either as

- intermediate-acting insulin (NPH or lente) at bedtime and in a small morning dose
- one or two daily injections of long-acting ultralente insulin, which in most patients is relatively peakless after steady state has been attained, or
- the basal component of a continuous subcutaneous insulin infusion (CSII) program.

Specific Flexible Multiple-Component Insulin Regimens

Premeal Regular and Basal Intermediate-Acting Insulins

This program uses three preprandial injections of regular insulin and intermediate-acting insulin (NPH or lente) given at bedtime to provide overnight basal insulinemia with peak serum insulin levels before breakfast (a time of a relative increase in insulin requirements and resistence known as the *dawn phenomenon)* (Fig. 6.2). Bedtime administration of intermediate-acting insulin also eliminates nocturnal peaks of insulin action, thus reducing risk of nocturnal hypoglycemia. A small morning dose of intermediate-acting insulin (perhaps 20–30% of the bedtime dose) provides daytime basal insulinemia and is used in most, but not all, patients. The intermediate-acting insulins are used this way quite effectively, because they have onset of action ~2 h after injection and produce peak insulin levels ~8–10 h after injection.

This program has become increasingly popular in recent years for a variety of reasons. It offers flexibility in meal size and timing. It is straightforward and easy to understand and implement, because each meal and each period of the day has a well-defined insulin component providing primary insulin action.

Premeal Regular and Basal Ultralente Insulin

This program uses three preprandial injections of regular insulin and long-acting ultralente insulin to provide basal insulinemia (Fig. 6.3). The ultralente insulin in most patients is relatively peakless after steady state has been attained.

This program originally was developed with beef or mixed beef-pork ultralente insulin preparations, which have a sluggish onset and an essentially flat action profile extending >36 h. Even with these insulins, many authorities divided the ultralente into two injections, administering half with the prebreakfast regular and half with the presupper regular insulin. This was to take advantage of the small peak in action seen in some patients 12–15 h after administration; it also limits the total volume of injection.

Human ultralente insulin has a broad peak ~10–16 h after injection and sustains its action up to 24 h and sometimes beyond. In most patients, the peak of human ultralente is sufficiently blunted at steady state to use as

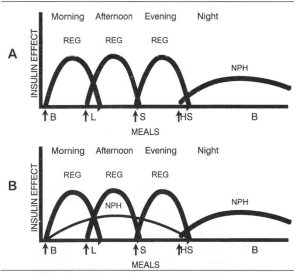

Fig. 6.2. Idealized Insulin Effect Provided by Multiple-Dose Regimens

A: preprandial injections of regular (REG) insulin before meals and basal intermediate-acting insulin (NPH or LENTE) at bedtime. **B:** preprandial injections of REG insulin before meals and basal regimen consisting of 2 daily injections of NPH or LENTE. *B*, breakfast; *L*, lunch; *S*, supper; *HS*, bedtime snack. *Arrows*, time of insulin injection, 30 min before meals.

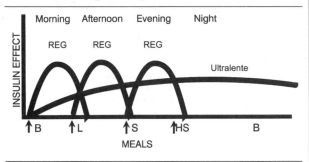

Fig. 6.3. Idealized Insulin Effect Provided by Multiple-Dose Regimen Providing Preprandial Injections of Regular (REG) Insulin Before Meals and Basal Long-Acting Ultralente Insulin

B, breakfast; *L,* lunch; *S,* supper; *HS,* bedtime snack. *Arrows,* time of insulin injection, 30 min before meals.

a *peakless* basal insulin. As a consequence of waning insulin effect around 24 h, there may be a rise in fasting glucose if human ultralente insulin is administered in a single morning dose. Thus, it probably is best to divide ultralente insulin into two doses (or to give it all in the evening, either before supper or at bedtime). There are some patients (usually thin individuals, *vide supra*) who appear to be *fast* absorbers of human insulin (both ultralente and intermediate-acting insulin). It may be desirable to use human ultralente as if it were an intermediate-acting insulin preparation in such individuals.

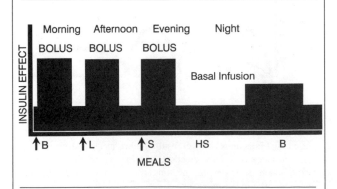

Fig. 6.4. Idealized Insulin Effect Provided by Continuous Subcutaneous Insulin Infusion

B, breakfast; *L,* lunch; *S,* supper; *HS,* bedtime snack.

Continuous Subcutaneous Insulin Infusion (See also INSULIN INFUSION PUMP THERAPY chapter.)

The most precise way to mimic normal insulin secretion clinically is to use an insulin pump in a program of CSII (Fig. 6.4). The pump delivers microliter amounts of regular insulin on a continual basis, thus replicating basal insulin secretion. Moreover, the basal rate may be programmed to vary at times of diurnal variation in insulin sensitivity, if it results in disruption of glycemic control. Thus, the basal infusion rate may be decreased overnight to avert nocturnal hypoglycemia or increased to counteract the dawn phenomenon, which often results in hyperglycemia on waking.

The pump may be activated before meals to provide increments of insulin as meal *boluses* or *boosts*. The meal insulin boluses are given ~20–30 min before a meal, whenever that meal is consumed. This allows total flexibility in meal timing. If a meal is skipped, the insulin bolus is omitted. If a meal is larger or smaller than usual, a larger or smaller insulin bolus is selected. Thus, patients on CSII have the potential of varying meal size and meal timing, as well as omitting meals, without sabotaging glycemic control.

Programmability also extends to the ability to *suspend* insulin delivery with increased physical activity, which reduces risk of exercise-related hypoglycemia. Patients should have syringes available for use any time there is interruption of insulin delivery, both for emergencies and for times that they may find the pump inconvenient (e.g., a day at the beach).

Other Intensive (But Less Flexible) Insulin Programs

Separate consideration of prandial and basal insulin needs permits flexibility in eating and activity. Yet, such an approach requires a motivated, educated patient who carefully monitors blood glucose several ($\geq$4) times daily. In the absence of either motivation, education, or frequent blood glucose monitoring, an alternative approach is to maintain day-to-day relative consistency of activity and timing and quantity of food intake, thus permitting prescription of a relatively constant insulin dose.

Split-and-Mixed Insulin Program
This program uses twice-daily administration of mixtures of regular insulin and intermediate-acting insulin (NPH or lente) (Fig. 6.5). Despite the development of more sophisticated and more physiologic insulin programs, the twice-daily split-and-mixed insulin schedule continues to enjoy popularity among doctors and patients and often receives much emphasis in the training of young physicians and medical students.

The advantage of this program is that it requires only two injections. Also, the doses of regular insulin before breakfast and supper may be increased or decreased for meals that are larger or smaller than average. Nevertheless, there are disadvantages that often preclude this program from being used in patients in whom the therapeutic goal is meticulous glycemic control. These disadvantages relate to the time-action profile of intermediate-acting insulin.

One problem concerns the daytime intermediate-acting insulin, given before breakfast to provide both daytime basal insulinemia and meal-related insulinemia for lunch. Because the intermediate-acting insulin has a broad peak, lunch and supper must be eaten on time to avoid hypoglycemia. Also, the peak effect of the insulin occurs 8–10 h after administration, too late to provide optimal insulin availability for lunch. Moreover, studies suggest that afternoon glycemia may be more dependent on morning regular rather than morning intermediate-acting insulin, contrary to traditional wisdom. Finally, because the intermediate-acting insulin is given before breakfast, it is difficult to make changes in the size or timing of lunch.

A more serious difficulty arises with the evening injection. Because intermediate-acting preparations produce peak insulin levels ~8–10 h after injection and wane thereafter, the

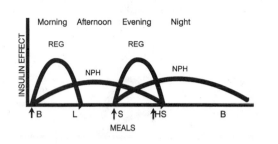

Fig. 6.5. Idealized Insulin Effect Provided by Insulin Regimen Consisting of 2 Daily Injections of Regular (REG) Insulin and Intermediate-Acting Insulin (NPH or LENTE)

B, breakfast; *L,* lunch; *S,* supper; *HS,* bedtime snack. *Arrows,* time of insulin injection, 30 min before meals.

effects of intermediate-acting insulin administered before supper may not be sustained throughout the night, resulting in morning hyperglycemia at a time of relatively increased insulin resistence and need, termed the *dawn phenomenon.* More importantly, attempts to correct this fasting hyperglycemia by increasing the dose often are complicated by nocturnal hypoglycemia when insulin action peaks.

Split-and-Mixed Program With Bedtime Intermediate Insulin
This program uses morning administration of a mixture of regular insulin and intermediate-acting insulin, with presupper regular insulin and bedtime intermediate-acting insulin, an approach used to minimize nocturnal hypoglycemia and to counteract the dawn phenomenon (Fig. 6.6). Taking intermediate-acting insulin at bedtime instead of before supper results in lower fasting and after-breakfast blood glucose levels.

The disadvantages of this program are that the patient still has little flexibility in meal schedule and the above problems related to daytime intermediate-acting insulin.

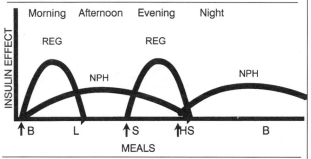

Fig. 6.6. Idealized Insulin Effect Provided by Insulin Regimen Consisting of a Morning Injection of Regular (REG) Insulin and Intermediate-Acting Insulin (NPH or LENTE), a Presupper Injection of Regular Insulin, and a Bedtime Injection of Intermediate-Acting Insulin

B, breakfast; *L,* lunch; *S,* supper; *HS,* bedtime snack. *Arrows,* time of insulin injection, 30 minutes before meals.

INSULIN DOSE AND DISTRIBUTION

Initial Insulin Doses

In typical patients with type I diabetes who are within 20% of their ideal body weight, in the absence of intercurrent infections or other periods of instability, the total daily insulin dose required for meticulous glycemic control is $0.5-1.0 \text{ U} \cdot \text{kg}^{-1}$ body wt $\cdot$ day^{-1}.

The required dose is less during the honeymoon period of relative remission early in the course of the disease (e.g., $0.2-0.6 \text{ U} \cdot \text{kg}^{-1} \cdot$ body wt $\cdot$ day^{-1}). Moreover, during the honeymoon period, because there is some continuing endogenous insulin secretion, it may be relatively easy to achieve glycemic control with virtually any rational insulin program.

During intercurrent illness, the insulin requirements may increase markedly (even double). Doses show progressive increases during pregnancy, increasing in units per kilogram. Because the patient's weight also increases, the total dose may even triple. Doses also increase during the adolescent growth spurt, and some adolescents have a sustained increased dose requirement.

Insulin Dose Distribution

About 40–50% of the total daily insulin dose is used to provide basal insulinemia. The remainder is divided among the meals either empirically, proportionate to the relative carbohydrate content of the meals, or by initially giving (in adults) ~0.8–1.2 U insulin for every 10 g carbohydrate consumed. Breakfast generally requires a slightly larger amount of insulin per 10 g carbohydrate than other meals.

Alternatively, a starting point for the initial distribution of insulin is
- basal 40–50% of total daily dose
- prebreakfast regular 15–25% of total daily dose
- prelunch regular ~15% of total daily dose, and
- presupper regular 15–20% of total daily dose.

Some patients desire or require a small dose of regular insulin to cover a bedtime snack (0–10% of daily total). Obviously, unusual meal distributions dictate a deviation from this scheme. Moreover, this dosage distribution is arbitrary and designed for an idealized average patient. Clearly, it must be individualized for any given patient, which is why it is best to base the premeal regular on meal content.

INSULIN ALGORITHMS

Patients are provided with an action plan to alter their therapy to achieve their individual, defined blood glucose targets. These actions are guided by SMBG determinations and daily records. The actions are a sequence of predetermined responses, a system of algorithms. The algorithms dictate that the patient intervene as necessary by altering insulin dosage, changing the timing of insulin injections in relation to meals, or changing the amount or content of food to be consumed.

Two general types of algorithms are used: *preprandial algorithms* and *pattern-adjustment algorithms.* The preprandial algorithms (also called *supplements)* provide an action plan that permits immediate action to be taken in response to current circumstances. The pattern-adjustment algorithms (also called *adjustments*) provide an action plan that permits corrective action to be taken when a recurrent pattern is seen in blood glucose fluctuations. Attainment of therapeutic goals requires that *both* types of algorithms be used.

Preprandial Algorithms

The preprandial algorithm action plan has been called a *scheme of insulin supplements* and a *sliding scale.* Because the actions taken may include changes in food intake and in timing of insulin administration, as well as changes in insulin dosage, the term *preprandial algorithm action plan* is preferable to *scheme of insulin supplements.* Many experts prefer to avoid the term *sliding scale,* because the traditional sliding scale used in many hospitals did not recognize ongoing (basal and prandial) insulin requirements and would prescribe no insulin when the blood glucose level was in the target range. The concept of supplements was introduced to emphasize that these changes in insulin dose were supplemental to the ongoing insulin requirements. Thus, insulin supplements are dosage variations to prevent or correct momentary deviations of blood glucose outside the target range. They may be used when there is variation in the quantity or pattern of meals or activities, when there is intercurrent illness or other stress, or when there is a need to correct variations in glycemia. Supplements, then, are temporary insulin doses. The use of supplements without pattern adjustment is not recommended and can lead to overinsulinization and weight gain. Conceptually, there are two types of supplements:
- **anticipatory supplements,** given to limit expected hyperglycemia, e.g., before a large meal, are used prospectively, and
- **compensatory supplements,** given in response to glycemic levels outside the target range, are used retrospectively.

Supplements may actually be decrements *(negative supplements),* e.g., lowering of preprandial regular insulin in anticipation of an unusually small meal or in the face of prevailing blood glucose levels lower than the preprandial target.

The preprandial algorithms provide an action plan for the patient guided by SMBG determinations and daily records. The actions depend on the answers to several questions that the patient asks at the time of any premeal insulin injection.
- What is my blood glucose now?
- What do I plan to eat now, i.e., usual size meal, large meal, or small meal, and how much carbohydrate?
- What do I plan to do after eating, i.e., usual activity, increased activity, or decreased activity?
- What has happened under these circumstances previously?

The answers dictate treatment response and become sensible routine decisions. The intervention actions dictated by the plan include food intake (altering the amount or content of food), activity, insulin dosage, and timing of injections in relation to meals. An example of a preprandialalgorithm action plan is shown in Table 6.2. The illustrative plan assumes that the preprandial and bedtime blood glucose target is 70–130 mg/dl (3.9–7.2 mM).

Pattern-Adjustment Algorithms

There should be a separate action plan used in response to a *pattern* of glycemia occurring over several days. These pattern-adjustment algorithms are small empirical changes made in the usual or basic insulin dosage, designed to gradually tailor, model, or shape the insulin dosage to the patient's usual or basic needs. In this sense, these algorithms are an ongoing iterative titration process based on experience.

The actions taken in the pattern-adjustment algorithms have been termed *insulin adjustments.* Thus, insulin *adjustments* are modifications in the usual or basic insulin dose, made in response to a *pattern* of glycemia.

Adustments are actions that presuppose that the patient has a relatively stable pattern of meals and activities,

---

Table 6.2. Sample Preprandial Action Plan

This action plan assumes that the preprandial blood glucose targets are 70–130 mg/dl (3.9–7.2 mM). Plans should be individualized for each patient. Once insulin dosage is stable and typical meal and activity patterns are established, use the following scheme for premeal alteration of dosage of regular insulin:

- **If blood glucose is <50 mg/dl (<2.8 mM):**
  - Reduce premeal regular insulin by 2–3 U.
  - Delay injection until immediately before eating.
  - Include at least 10 g carbohydrate in the meal.
- **If blood glucose is 50–70 mg/dl (2.8–3.9 mM):**
  - Reduce premeal regular insulin by 1–2 U.
  - Delay injection until immediately before eating.
- **If blood glucose is 70–130 mg/dl (3.9–7.2 mM):**
  - Take prescribed premeal dose of regular insulin.
- **If blood glucose is 130–150 mg/dl (7.2–8.3 mM):**
  - Increase premeal dose of regular insulin by 1 U.
- **If blood glucose is 150–200 mg/dl (8.3–11.1 mM):**
  - Increase premeal dose of regular insulin by 2 U.
- **If blood glucose is 200–250 mg/dl (11.1–13.9 mM):**
  - Increase premeal dose of regular insulin by 3 U.
  - Consider delaying the meal an extra 15 min (to 45 min after injection).
- **If blood glucose is 250–300 mg/dl (13.9–16.7 mM):**
  - Increase premeal dosage of regular insulin by 4 U.
  - Consider delaying the meal an extra 20–30 min (to 40–60 min after injection).
- **If blood glucose is 300–350 mg/dl (16.7–19.4 mM):**
  - Increase premeal dosage of regular insulin by 5 U.

- Delay meal an extra 20–30 min (to 40–60 min after injection).
- Check urine ketones. If the amount is moderate to large, increase fluid intake and consider extra insulin (1–2 U). Recheck blood glucose and urine ketones in 2–3 h.
- **If blood glucose is 350–400 mg/dl (19.4–22.2 mM):**
  - Increase premeal dosage of regular insulin by 6 U.
  - Delay meal an extra 20–30 min (to 40–60 min after injection).
  - Check urine ketones. If the amount is moderate to large, increase fluid intake and consider extra insulin (1–2 U). Recheck blood glucose and urine ketones in 2–3 h.
- **If blood glucose is >400 mg/dl (>22.2 mM):**
  - Increase premeal dosage of regular insulin by 7 U.
  - Delay meal an extra 30 min (to 50–60 min after injection).
  - Check urine ketones. If the amount is moderate to large, increase fluid intake and consider extra insulin (1–2 U). Recheck blood glucose and urine ketones in 2–3 h.
- **If planned meal is larger than usual:**
  - Increase regular insulin by 1–2 U.
- **If planned meal is smaller than usual:**
  - Decrease regular insulin by 1–2 U.
- **If unusual, increased activity is planned after eating:**
  - Eat extra carbohydrate and/or decrease regular insulin by 1–2 U.
- **If unusual, sedentary activity is planned after eating:**
  - Consider increasing regular insulin by 1–2 U.

Table 6.3. Sample Pattern-Adjustment Action Plan

This action plan assumes that the preprandial blood glucose targets are 70–130 mg/dl (3.9–7.2 mM). Plans should be individualized for each patient.

- *Assumptions*
  - Basal insulin (bedtime intermediate-acting NPH insulin, ultralente insulin, or basal rate of insulin pump) is the major insulin acting overnight. Its effect is reflected in the results of blood glucose tests during the middle of the night and on arising the next morning.
  - Prebreakfast regular insulin has its major action between breakfast and lunch. Its effect is primarily reflected in the results of blood glucose tests before lunch.
  - Prelunch regular insulin has its major action between lunch and supper. Its effect is primarily reflected in the results of blood glucose tests before supper.
  - Presupper regular insulin has its major action between

- *Hyperglycemia not explained by unusual diet/exercise/insulin*
  - If prebreakfast blood glucose is >130 mg/dl (>7.2 mM) for 3–5 days in a row, increase basal insulin (bedtime NPH or ultralente) by 1 or 2 U (0.05–0.1 U/h for CSII). (Before making such changes, verify that the blood glucose nadir, usually around 0200–0400, is not <70 mg/dl [<3.9 mM].)
  - If prelunch blood glucose is >130 mg/dl (>7.2 mM) for 3–5 days in a row, increase prebreakfast regular insulin by 1 or 2 U.
  - If presupper blood glucose is >130 mg/dl (>7.2 mM) for 3–5 days in a row, increase prelunch regular insulin by 1 or

2 U.
  - If bedtime blood glucose is (>130 mg/dl (>7.2 mM) for 3–5 days in a row, increase presupper regular insulin by 1 or 2 U.
  - Only increase one insulin component at a time, starting with the one affecting the earliest blood glucose during the day.

- *Hypoglycemia not explained by unusual diet/exercise/insulin*
  - If prebreakfast blood glucose is <70 mg/dl (<3.9 mM), or if there is evidence of hypoglycemic reactions occurring during the night, reduce basal insulin (bedtime NPH or ultralente) by 1 or 2 U (0.05–0.1 U/h for CSII).
  - If prelunch blood glucose is <70 mg/dl (<3.9 mM), or if you have a hypoglycemic reaction between breakfast and lunch, reduce prebreakfast regular insulin by 1 or 2 U.
  - If presupper blood glucose is <70 mg/dl (<3.9 mM), or if you have a hypoglycemic reaction between lunch and supper, reduce prelunch regular insulin by 1 or 2 U.
  - If bedtime blood glucose is <70 mg/dl (<3.9 mM), or if you have a hypoglycemic reaction between supper and bedtime, reduce presupper regular insulin by 1 or 2 U.
  - Verify hypoglycemic symptoms with blood glucose measurements. Treat hypoglycemic reactions with 10–15 g carbohydrate.

has no intercurrent illness, and is free from unusual stress.

Pattern-adjustment algorithms provide that when the blood glucose is consistently above or below the target range at a particular time day, a pattern has been established and action must be taken. The action is that the insulin dose (of the relevant insulin component most likely responsible) must be either increased or decreased to correct the pattern of glycemia outside the target range. The continuing need for preprandial actions (e.g., compensatory insulin supplements) to correct unexplained ambient glycemia outside the target range at a particular time of the day indicates that an adjustment should be made in the relevant insulin component. Pattern-adjustment algorithms provide for prospective changes based on retrospective data. They are not dependent on the blood glucose at the moment when they are implemented. Instead, they anticipate insulin need for the next time period. An example of a pattern-adjustment algorithm action plan is shown in Table 6.3 for an insulin program involving preprandial regular insulin and bedtime intermediate-acting insulin.

INJECTION DEVICES

Making insulin injections easier and more comfortable assists patients in complying with a treatment plan. In particular, patients may be more open to initiating intensive diabetes management if taking multiple daily insulin injections is made as convenient as possible.

With **spring-loaded devices,** the patient places a conventional insulin syringe in the device, activates it, and allows the device to inject the insulin.

Jet injection devices supply a subcutaneous spray of insulin that is forced under high pressure using compressed air. These devices are bulkier than conventional syringes but do not use a needle and may be less painful. When jet injection devices are used properly, the level of free insulin is comparable to that achieved with a conventional needle and syringe. Jet administration results in more rapid absorption of insulin, and blood glucose levels are well controlled. To be effective, however, the device must be set for optimal penetration, which varies among individuals and can vary within an individual depending on the injection site and the dose. Jet injectors must be cleaned properly every 2 wk and are somewhat more complicated to use than a conventional syringe.

Insulin pens are especially useful in intensive insulin therapy. Insulin cartridges containing 150 U of either regular, NPH, or 70/30 insulin are placed in a pen-like device. Disposable needles are attached to the end of the insulin pen. The desired dose is administered by turning a dial selector and pushing a button at the end of the insulin pen. Insulin pens are convenient to carry in a pocket, purse, or briefcase; make insulin injections easy to administer outside the home; and eliminate the need to draw up insulin frequently throughout the day.

Injection port is the term used to describe small needles or Teflon catheters with an external port can be inserted into the abdomen or other subcutaneous tissue and remain in place for several days. Injections can be given through the catheter, instead of through the skin, thus minimizing needle punctures.

BIBLIOGRAPHY

Hirsch IB, Farkas–Hirsch R, Skyler JS: Intensive insulin therapy for treatment of type I diabetes. *Diabetes Care* 13:1265–83, 1990

Howorka K: *Functional Insulin Treatment.* Berlin, Springer–Verlag, 1990

Nolte MS: Insulin therapy in insulin–dependent (type I) diabetes mellitus: *Endocrin Metab Clin North Am* 21:281–312, 1992

Schade DS, Santiago JV, Skyler JS, Rizza R: *Intensive Insulin Therapy.* Princeton, NJ, Excerpta Med., 1983

Insulin Infusion Pump Therapy

Highlights

Why Use CSII?

Insulin Dosage Calculations for Insulin Pump Therapy

Insulin Adjustments
    Diet
    Exercise
    Illness
    Correction of Hyperglycemia

Risks of CSII
    Skin Infection
    Unexplained Hyperglycemia
    Hypoglycemia

Wearing the Pump

Patient Education for CSII

Implantable Insulin Infusion Pumps

Highlights
Insulin Infusion Pump Therapy

- Insulin therapy by an insulin infusion pump closely approximates normal physiological insulin delivery by continuously delivering a basal rate of rapid-acting insulin and allowing bolus insulin administration before meals.

- For the motivated and capable patient with the necessary resources, insulin pump therapy is indicated for
  - suboptimal glycemic control
  - wide blood glucose excursions
  - dawn phenomenon with elevated fasting blood glucose levels
  - nocturnal hypoglycemia
  - frequent severe hypoglycemia
  - pregnancy or planned pregnancy
  - day-to-day variations in schedule that are not well managed by multiple insulin injections.

- Basal rate should consist of 40-60% of the patient's total daily insulin dose. Several basal rates can be set in a 24-h period to accommodate diurnal variations in insulin sensitivity.

- Meal boluses can be calculated based on carbohydrate content, using a ratio of 1 U insulin/10-15 g carbohydrate, or with a formula based on a percentage of the total daily dose, e.g., breakfast, 20%; lunch, 10%; dinner, 15%; and bedtime, 5%. In addition, insulin algorithms can be devised to assist patients in adjusting boluses based on premeal blood glucose levels.

- Patients can be taught to make additional adjustments in the basal rate and/or bolus size for illness, exercise, and between-meal hyperglycemia.

- Risks of insulin pump therapy include
  - skin infections, which can be avoided or resolved with regular changes of the infusion set, by keeping the infusion site clean and dry, and by removing the infusion set at the first signs of discomfort or redness
  - unexplained hyperglycemia, which usually results from a partial or complete interruption of insulin delivery, and
  - hypoglycemia, which can be minimized by monitoring blood glucose levels at least four times per day, weekly at 0300, and before operating a motor vehicle.

- The insulin pump should be worn at all times. The patient should use an alternate insulin regimen if the pump is removed for more than 1-2 h.

- Successful insulin pump therapy requires thorough and ongoing education in technical components of the insulin pump and skills needed to adjust insulin for variations in daily activities.

- Implantable insulin pumps are experimental and not commercially available in the U.S.

Insulin Infusion Pump Therapy

The search for optimal insulin regimens has led to the development of technology that facilitates physiological insulin replacement and patient compliance to treatment recommendations. Insulin infusion pumps deliver insulin continuously in a manner that approximates normal physiological insulin delivery and provide flexibility in day-to-day diabetes management. Along with blood glucose self-monitoring, insulin pumps make near-physiological insulin delivery possible for patients with diabetes to achieve near-normoglycemia.

Continuous subcutaneous insulin infusion (CSII) involves the use of a small pump or mechanical device into which a reservoir or syringe that contains regular insulin is placed. This syringe is connected to a 24- or 42-inch length of plastic tubing. At the end of the tubing is a 27-gauge needle or a soft Teflon cannula that the patient inserts into the subcutaneous tissue. The usual site of injection is the abdomen because insulin absorption is most consistent from this site and patients find placement of the needle in the abdomen simple and comfortable. After the syringe is placed in the pump, a mechanism, such as a lead screw, advances the plunger of the syringe, delivering insulin continuously into the patient according to the rate(s) programmed into the pump.

Insulin is delivered by the insulin pump in two ways. Basal insulin delivery is the continuous infusion of insulin and usually ranges from 0.4 to 2.0 U/h. Insulin pumps can be programmed to give up to 6, or as many as 24, different basal rates in a given 24-h period, depending on the pump used. Most patients achieve glycemic goals using 1–2 basal rates over a 24-h period. Insulin is also delivered as a bolus, or larger amount of insulin, given at a distinct time in anticipation of a meal. The bolus infusion is programmed and administered when bolus delivery is desired. The bolus mode also can be used to correct hyperglycemia that may result from illness, stress, or increased dietary intake.

Insulin infusion pumps have therapeutic and safety features that facilitate the achievement of treatment goals in various situations.

- Adjustments in the basal rate can be made temporarily for periods of increased activity, illness, or stress without changing the usual basal rate program.
- Basal delivery can be suspended if necessary.
- Bolus doses and the time of their delivery can be reviewed.
- Total daily insulin delivery can be monitored. Insulin pumps can be programmed to deliver U-40, U-50, or U-100 insulin, depending on the model used.
- There are alarm systems for low battery, empty syringe, occlusion, and electronic malfunction.

WHY USE CSII?

The benefits of CSII therapy are derived from the pharmacologic advantage of using only rapid-acting insulin that is delivered as a continuous infusion, with incremental bolus administration at meals. This mode of insulin delivery most closely approximates physiologic delivery. It also minimizes depots of insulin characteristic of conventional insulin delivery via syringe that can be mobilized by increased blood flow associated with exercise or warm baths. Rapid-acting insulin is associated with the least amount of variation in day-to-day absorption. Because of the basal infusion, premeal boluses of insulin need not be given until ~20–30 min before the meal is consumed. In addition, meals can be skipped, delayed, or altered without loss of glycemic control.

Basal infusions can be programmed to coincide with the diurnal variation of insulin sensitivity and requirements. Patients often need lower basal rates during the night (~2300 to 0400) and higher basal rates between 0300 or 0400 and 0900 to deal with the dawn phenomenon. Temporary basal rate adjustments can be made during exercise, during the postexercise period when hypoglycemia is likely to occur, or during illness when insulin requirements tend to be higher.

Thus, insulin pump therapy optimizes the conditions for achieving good glycemic control while maintaining lifestyle flexibility. This therapeutic approach provides patients with the opportunity to fully participate in their self-care, because decisions and adjustments about aspects of the regimen can be made on a moment-to-moment basis as aspects of daily life are encountered.

Because of these characteristics, patients should be considered for insulin pump therapy

- to improve or stabilize glycemic control, especially if multiple daily insulin regimens have failed to solve self-management problems such as wide glycemic excursions, nocturnal hypoglycemia, and effects of the dawn phenomenon
- to increase lifestyle flexibility and deal with day-to-day variations in work or exercise schedule, and/or
- to meet increased self-management needs, i.e., to allow greater participation in self-care.

Patients who have erratic schedules, work different shifts, or travel extensively can benefit greatly from insulin pump therapy.

INITIAL DOSAGE CALCULATIONS FOR INSULIN PUMP THERAPY

The total 24-h basal rate is usually 40–50% of the patient's total daily dose. The meal boluses can be calculated as a percentage of the total daily dose as follows:

- breakfast, 20%,
- lunch, 10%,
- dinner, 15%, and
- bedtime, 5%.

Alternatively, meal boluses can be matched to the patient's intake of carbohydrate at each meal with a ratio of ~1U/10–15 g carbohydrate. The bedtime bolus is optional depending on the patient's bedtime blood glucose level and desire or need for a bedtime snack.

Generally, the basal rate should be no more than 60% of the patient's total daily dose. If the patient has reasonably good glycemic control, the prepump total daily dose may need to be reduced by 10% before calculating pump dosages because insulin requirements may decrease with insulin pump therapy.

For example, a patient who is taking 22 U NPH insulin and 8 U regular insulin before breakfast and 10 U NPH and 6 U regular before dinner, for a total daily dose of 46 U, would be started on the following insulin schedule for the pump:

- basal rate:
$$\frac{46 \times 50\% \ (0.5 \times 46)}{24 \ h} = 1 \ U/h$$
- boluses
  - breakfast, 9 U (46 x 0.2 or 20%)
  - lunch, 4.5 U (46 x 0.1 or 10%)
  - dinner, 7 U (46 x 0.15 or 15%)
  - bedtime, 2 U (46 x 0.5 or 5%).

An alternate method to calculate the total daily basal rate is to multiply the patient's weight in kilograms by 0.3. If the patient's weight was 80 kg (176 lb), the basal rate would be

$$\frac{80 \times 0.3}{24 \ h} = 1 \ U/h$$

Assuming that the basal rate was 50% of the total daily dose, the boluses would be calculated as above, using 48 U as the total daily dose.

Most patients require basal rates that fall within the range of 0.4–2.U/h, with the average basal rate being 0.7–0.9 U/h. Average adults require $0.5–1.0 \ U \cdot kg^{-1}$ body wt $\cdot day^{-1}$.

Patients using insulin pump therapy have the advantage of programming different basal rates for varying diurnal insulin needs. Patients often need lower basal rates between bedtime and 0300–0500, and higher basal rates between 0300–0900 to deal with the dawn phenomenon. An intermediate basal rate may be needed during the rest of the day. An adjustment of the basal rate by 10–20% is usually recommended. Using the example above, if the patient's blood glucose profile indicated that these varying diurnal insulin needs were evident, the basal rate profile might be

- 2300–0300, 0.9 U/h
- 0300–0700, 1.2 U/h, and
- 0700–2300, 1.0 U/h.

After calculating insulin boluses using the above formula, evaluate these dosages relative to the patient's prescribed meal plan. An average of 1 U of regular insulin will cover 10–15 g carbohydrate, with a range of 0.5–2.0 U. For a meal containing 60 g carbohydrate, a bolus dose of 4–6 U would be a reasonable start. The 9-U breakfast bolus calculated above (20% of the total daily dose of 46 U) would probably be too much for a 60-g carbohydrate meal. Therefore, a lower starting bolus of insulin at breakfast may be indicated.

As with all insulin regimens and insulin adjustments, careful blood glucose monitoring must be performed to determine the effectiveness of insulin dosages relative to a meal plan and to the patient's usual activity level. Blood glucose testing should be done initially 30 min before each meal, 90–120 min after each meal, at bedtime, and at 0300 until glycemic goals are achieved. Further adjustments will be required as the patient implements the insulin regimen under various situations. A minimum of premeal, bedtime, and weekly 0300 blood glucose testing should be performed.

The premeal boluses should be adjusted based on the postprandial and next premeal blood glucose level. For example, if the blood glucose levels 1.5–2.0 h after breakfast and before lunch are higher than desired, the pre-breakfast bolus should be increased by 1–2 U.

Evaluate the basal rate by the 0300 and fasting blood glucose levels. If these values are higher or lower than desired, the basal rate should be adjusted accordingly, usually by increments of 0.1–0.2 U/h. If the 0300 and fasting blood glucose levels are widely discrepant, then different basal rates may be needed during sleep and in the early morning (before waking) hours. Adjust the daytime basal rate based on the blood glucose levels that occur when meals are skipped or delayed. For example, if the patient becomes hypoglycemic when meals are skipped or delayed, the daytime basal rate is too high.

Insulin algorithms provide patients with a means to adjust premeal boluses based on premeal blood glucose levels. The algorithm in Table 7.1 assumes that a patient requires 1 U regular insulin for every 50 mg/dl (2.8 mM) blood glucose. Typically, patients require ~1 U for every 40–50 mg/dl (2.2–2.8 mM) blood glucose, but this varies depending on the patient's insulin sensitivity and daily insulin requirements. For example, a patient taking 20 U insulin/day may

Table 7.1. Sample Variable Insulin Dosage Schedule for Insulin Infusion Pump Therapy (Regular Insulin Only)*

BLOOD GLUCOSE		UNITS OF INSULIN			
mg/dl	mM	BREAKFAST	LUNCH	SUPPER	BEDTIME SNACK
<70	<3.9	4	3	5	0
71–100	3.9–5.5	6	4	6	0
101–150	5.6–8.3	8	5	7	1
151–200	8.4–11.1	9	6	8	2
201–250	11.2–13.0	10	7	9	2
251–300	13.9–16.7	11	9	11	3
>300	>16.7	12	10	13	4

*Basal rate = 1.0 U/h

require only 0.5 U insulin for every 50 mg/dl (2.8 mM) blood glucose, whereas, a patient taking 80 U insulin/day may require 2–3 U insulin for every 50 mg/dl (2.8 mM) blood glucose.

The timing of the premeal insulin bolus also can be varied depending on the premeal blood glucose level. The insulin bolus should be given 20–30 min before ingesting a meal. Increasing this time to 45–60 min can improve insulin effectiveness, especially if the premeal blood glucose level is elevated.

INSULIN ADJUSTMENTS

Diet

Patients can be taught to adjust insulin boluses for variations in dietary intake, so that blood glucose levels remain in the desired range. Usually 1 U insulin will cover 10–15 g carbohydrate. However, this can range from 0.5 to 2.0 U/10–15 g carbohydrate and can vary depending on the time of the meal (i.e., generally, more insulin is required at breakfast, less at lunch, and an intermediate amount at dinner). More precise estimates of the patient's insulin needs can be determined.

Exercise

Premeal regular insulin can be decreased 25–50% for moderate levels of planned postprandial activity. If the activity is strenuous, additional carbohydrate may also be needed. A temporary reduction in the basal rate of 20–40% may be necessary for sustained periods of exercise lasting >60 min. A temporary 25% reduction in the basal rate during postexercise hours may be necessary to avoid postexercise hypoglycemia. Suspending the basal rate for >1–2 h is not recommended. Activities such as yard work, shopping, and housework are common events that frequently result in episodes of hypoglycemia. A reduction in insulin for these kinds of activities is also required.

If the patient engages in unplanned exercise, additional carbohydrate must be consumed (see NUTRITIONAL MANAGEMENT).

Illness

The insulin pump facilitates managing blood glucose levels during periods of illness, especially when patients must significantly modify their food intake. A 20–50% increase in the basal rate and/or premeal boluses is usually needed to accommodate increased insulin requirements during illness. The basal rate should be adjusted so that blood glucose levels remain in a desired range overnight and during the day when meals are delayed or not eaten with regularity because of the illness. Boluses can be adjusted to the patient's calorie intake. Frequent blood glucose and urine ketone monitoring should be performed.

Correction of Hyperglycemia

Supplemental insulin can be taken when the patient wishes to correct hyperglycemia in the absence of any food intake. This supplemental insulin should not be confused with the insulin adjustment shown in Table 7.1 for varying blood glucose levels before a meal. The bolus mode of the pump can be used at any time simply to correct postprandial hyperglycemia or any hyperglycemia that occurs as a result of some change in routine or error in judgment about an adjustment made for food or exercise. Generally, 1 U insulin will lower blood glucose by 50–100 mg/dl (2.8–5.6 mM). A conservative approach is to have the patient take 1 U insulin to lower an elevated blood glucose level by 100 mg/dl (5.6 mM). If blood glucose testing reveals that this is not an adequate amount of insulin, the patient can use a 1-U supplemental insulin dose to lower the blood glucose by 75 mg/dl (4.2 mM), and so on. For example, if a patient obtains a blood glucose reading of 243 mg/dl (13.5 mM) 2 h after a restaurant meal, he or she can take a 1- to 2-U bolus to lower blood glucose to the desired range (<180 mg/dl [<10 mM]). When determining the amount of supplemental insulin, the patient should be advised to consider the time of the last bolus. If the last bolus was taken <4 h ago, some percentage of activity from that bolus remains; therefore, the supplemental insulin dose should be reduced with that in mind.

RISKS OF CSII

Skin Infection

Skin infections can occur at the infusion site. These infections can range from a small area of mild inflammation and tenderness to a large area of induration, inflammation, and soreness with purulent drainage. Antibiotics usually resolve these infections completely. Large abscesses may have to be surgically incised and drained.

To avoid infections, the infusion site should be kept clean and dry at all times. Soap and water usually are adequate to cleanse the skin before needle insertion. Antibacterial cleansers may be needed for patients who experience recurrent infusion site infections. Known carriers of *Staphylococcus aureus* require antibacterial cleansers and meticulous care of the infusion site and may benefit from antibiotic treatment. Patients should be instructed to remove moist tape and to clean and dry the area around the needle insertion site. This procedure is important during the summer or during increased physical activity.

The infusion set should be removed every 24–72 h and should not be reused. Subsequent infusion sites should be at least 1-inch apart at various locations around the abdomen. The needle should be comfortable at all times and removed immediately if irritation, redness, or inflammation occur. The infusion set should not be placed at the belt line or where constrictive clothing will cause additional irritation. Skin–Prep, a protective dressing for sensitive skin, can be applied to the skin before taping the infusion set in place. Skin Tac, a liquid adhesive, also can be brushed onto the skin before applying tape to help the tape adhere better. If any redness persists or worsens, the health–care provider should be notified within 24 h.

Patients sometimes report that insertion of the infusion set is difficult and/or that blood glucose levels are higher when the infusion set is placed in areas with scar tissue or where underlying tissue feels hard or tough. These areas should be avoided because insulin absorption may be poor or unpredictable. Alternative sites, such as the hip or thigh, can be used until the tissue has healed.

There are several types of infusion sets with various catheter and needle types: 24- and 42-inch lengths are available with straight or angled needles, needles attached to an adhesive disk, and Teflon catheters with needle introducers. Infusion sets with a quick-release feature that allows the patient to disconnect easily from the pump without removing the syringe or infusion set will soon be available. Most catheter or infusion site problems, such as difficulty with needle insertion and skin breakdown, can be resolved by finding the type of catheter and tape that meets the patient's needs. Tegaderm, Polyskin, or any surgical tape can be used to secure the needle and catheter in place. Consult the pump manufacturer for specific product information.

Unexplained Hyperglycemia

Because the insulin pump uses regular insulin only, even a partial interruption of insulin delivery can result in hyperglycemia. Complete interruption of insulin delivery can result in ketosis or ketoacidosis in a matter of hours.

Patients new to insulin pump therapy must be taught to consider the possibility of interrupted insulin delivery any time high blood glucose levels persist for no apparent reason. In the absence of illness, if there has been no increase in dietary intake, no change in the insulin dose or timing, or no alteration in stress or activity levels, a disruption in insulin delivery should be suspected if hyperglycemia persists. The first indication of unexplained hyperglycemia often occurs with a routine blood glucose test, when the patient is surprised by an unusually high reading. If the blood glucose level has not decreased 2–4 h later, especially if an additional bolus of insulin has been taken, hyperglycemia caused by some interruption of insulin delivery is the likely cause. If urine ketones

are present also, a serious disruption of insulin delivery must be considered.

There are many potential causes of unexplained hyperglycemia or ketoacidosis related to partial or complete failure of some component of the insulin infusion pump/syringe/infusion set system (Table 7.2). When a patient encounters a high blood glucose level (>250 mg/dl [>13.8 mM]) that cannot be explained by an alteration in a component of the treatment plan, a systematic investigation of the pump, syringe, infusion set, infusion site, and insulin should be performed to identify the cause.

- If the patient detects a problem with the site, the infusion set tubing, or the connection between the syringe and the infusion set, then the catheter and site should be changed.
- If a problem with the pump is identified, the pump should be reprogrammed or replaced.
- If the syringe or insulin is faulty, the insulin, syringe, infusion set, and site should be changed.

If no obvious cause is found, the patient should assume that there is an infusion problem, most likely caused by a partial or complete occlusion of insulin in the infusion set or at the infusion site. If this is the case, the syringe, insulin, infusion set, and site should be replaced. Sometimes the insulin itself loses potency over time, and simply using a new bottle of insulin will correct the problem.

If the pump is inoperable or malfunctioning, a multiple-injection regimen should be used until the pump can be replaced. All patients should know how to use an alternative insulin regimen with conventional insulin syringes, in case a problem with the pump or some component of the infusion system occurs. The patient must be instructed to always carry extra insulin, pump supplies (batteries, infusion sets, and pump syringes), and conventional syringes. If a pump malfunction is suspected, the health-care provider should be contacted. Also, assistance can be obtained from the technical services of the pump manufacturer.

Table 7.2. Unexplained Hyperglycemia: Factors to Consider

- Insulin pump
  - Basal rate programmed incorrectly
  - Battery depleted
  - Pump malfunction
  - Syringe does not advance properly
  - Program/pump alarms
  - Program functions cannot be set
- Syringe
  - Improper placement in the pump
  - Empty syringe (insulin depleted)
  - Leakage of insulin
  - Syringe not primed
- Infusion set/needle
  - Insulin leakage
  - Dislodged needle
  - Air in infusion set
  - Blood in infusion set
  - High-pressure alarm
  - Type of infusion set may not be insulin compatible
  - Infusion set in place >48 h
  - Kink in the tubing
  - Occlusion of the insulin
  - Loose syringe/infusion set connection
- Infusion site
  - Redness, irritation, inflammation, induration
  - Discomfort
  - Placement in the area of hypertrophy or scar tissue
  - Placement in the area of friction or near the belt line
- Insulin
  - Insulin is not buffered
  - Insulin has clumped particles or crystallized appearance
  - Insulin is beyond expiration date
  - Insulin was exposed to temperature extremes
  - Insulin vial has been used for >1 mo or is nearly empty

When unexplained hyperglycemia is detected and the source of the problem is corrected, then the hyperglycemia and ketonuria must be treated. Blood glucose and urine ketone levels should be monitored every 2–3 h; insulin boluses should be taken in amounts determined by the patient's insulin sensitivity and daily insulin requirements until urine ketones have cleared and blood glucose levels have returned to the desired range. Insulin may need to be taken via conventional injections to correct the hyperglycemia and ketosis, especially if pump malfunction is suspected.

The incidence of unexplained hyperglycemia can be reduced by following a few guidelines. The use of buffered insulin and infusion sets that are lined with insulin-compatible material (Minimed Technologies Polyfin and Sof-Set) can help prevent insulin precipitation and clogging. If the basal rates are <0.6 U/h, diluting the insulin to U-40 or U-50 may be necessary to minimize the formation of occlusions. Diluent can be obtained from the insulin manufacturer. Infusion sets should be changed at least every 24–72 h. If blood appears in the tubing, the infusion set should be replaced immediately, because the blood may clot and block insulin delivery. Ideally, infusion sets should be inserted before the administration of a bolus to lessen the possibility that tissue will clog the needle. The infusion set should not be inserted into scar tissue or into tissue that is hardened or tough. Ketosis and/or ketoacidosis can be completely avoided if patients monitor blood glucose levels frequently and correct unexplained hyperglycemia as soon as it occurs.

Hypoglycemia

The frequency of hypoglycemia does not seem to be significantly greater with insulin pump therapy compared to multiple daily insulin injections. Hypoglycemia is more likely related to errors in self-management, attempts to achieve normoglycemia, and impaired glucose counterregulation. Strategies for avoiding and methods of teaching hypoglycemia are essentially the same for any intensive diabetes management approach, regardless of the mode of insulin therapy. Family members should know how to suspend pump operation in the event of severe hypoglycemia.

Avoiding severe hypoglycemia begins with insulin pump use by patients who are good candidates for intensive therapy (Table 7.3). Patients must be prepared to check blood glucose levels at least four times a day to monitor pump operation and to make and evaluate decisions regarding insulin doses. Physical capabilities to program the pump and monitor its operation are necessary; patients must be able to understand the relationships between components of the treatment plan and their effects on blood glucose levels. Anticipating insulin needs for varying activities increases the likelihood that appropriate adjustments in insulin will be made and that blood glucose levels will remain in the desired range.

WEARING THE PUMP

The pump needs to be worn at all times. Removal of the pump for >1–2 h without insulin compensation puts the patient at risk for developing hyperglycemia and ketosis. Patients are frequently concerned about initiating insulin pump therapy because they believe that it will interfere with activities they enjoy. The pump can be worn during most activities, with the possible exception of strenuous contact sports. Pumps are small enough to be worn on a belt, in a pants or shirt pocket, or clipped to underclothing. During sleep, pumps usually are placed next to the wearer or under the pillow. With 42 inches of infusion set tubing, movement is relatively unrestricted. During sexual activity, a garter is an alternative for women to secure the pump. If the pump is not waterproof, it must be removed for showering or placed in a plastic sheath (the Shower-Pak). Water sports also would require removal of the pump or placement of the pump in a waterproof holder (the Sportsguard).

Most patients are concerned about what to do with the insulin pump during sexual activity, but they may not feel comfortable asking about it. If the patient does not bring up the topic, the

---

Table 7.3. Patient Selection Criteria for Insulin Pump Use

- Medical/metabolic indications
  - Suboptimal glycemic control
  - Wide blood glucose excursions
  - Dawn phenomenon with elevated fasting blood glucose levels
  - Frequent severe hypoglycemia
  - Nocturnal hypoglycemia
  - Pregnant or planning conception
  - Variable daily schedule not well managed with injections
- Technical/physical ability
  - Perform blood glucose monitoring accurately and frequently
  - Perform the technical components of insulin pump use
  - Ensure the absence of serious disease or disability that would impair technical performance
- Intellectual ability
  - Learn the technical and cognitive components of pump use, e.g., meal planning, the meaning of blood glucose levels, adjusting insulin
  - Determine the relationship between aspects of the regimen, e.g., food and insulin, activity and blood glucose levels
  - Determine the relationship between behavior and outcome (actions and results)
  - Change behavior or aspects of the regimen based on the evaluation of outcomes
- Motivational ability
  - Perform frequent blood glucose monitoring
  - Comply with recommendations for safe insulin pump use
  - Pay attention to aspects of daily life as they affect the insulin regimen and the needed adjustments
  - Anticipate insulin needs as circumstances change
  - Evaluate actions taken; engage in problem-solving behavior
- Financial resources
  - Has a source of reimbursement for insulin pump and blood glucose monitoring supplies and ongoing health care

---

health-care provider should initiate a discussion about sexual activity and pump use. Most couples find that wearing the insulin pump during sexual activity does not interfere with sexual intimacy. If the pump is disconnected during sexual activity, the patient should be cautioned to resume insulin pump delivery within an hour or so. After sexual activity, the tape and infusion set should be checked to ensure that the system is intact and secure.

There are alternatives for patients who do not wish to wear their pumps for certain periods of time, including days at the beach, vacations, or an evening out.

- The infusion set can be clamped and disconnected from the pump for up to 1–2 h depending on the level of activity. The needle is left in place in the abdomen.
- The patient can take injections of regular insulin before meals and wear the pump at night to provide basal insulin needs.
- A multiple daily injection regimen of premeal regular insulin and bedtime NPH or lente insulin can be used until pump therapy is resumed.
- The premeal regular insulin dosage should be 40–50% more than is prescribed during pump use. This compensates for the missing basal insulin infusion. The NPH insulin used to provide for insulin needs overnight should be ~70–80% of the usual total amount of basal insulin taken in 24 h, or 1.5–2.0 times the amount of basal insulin usually received overnight.

Patients need to be reminded that there are some limitations on the timing of insulin and meals while off the pump. More blood glucose monitoring should be performed while using an alternative insulin regimen.

PATIENT EDUCATION FOR CSII

Appropriate education for insulin pump therapy takes place in four phases (Table 7.4). The first phase occurs before initiating pump therapy. During this period, the advantages and disadvantages of pump therapy are discussed, the patient's treatment goals relative to pump therapy are reviewed, and the patient's resources to successfully manage insulin pump therapy are identified. Strategies to establish the patient's suitability for insulin pump use can be initiated. A trial of performing and recording four blood glucose tests per day, using a multiple daily insulin regimen or insulin algorithms with an existing insulin regimen, can be used.

Once a decision to initiate insulin pump therapy is made, the second phase of education begins. During this period, the patient is taught the technical components of using the insulin pump (Table 7.5). Blood glucose testing skills are verified, meal planning is taught or reviewed, and pump therapy is initiated. This education can be accomplished through a series of outpatient visits with the nurse specialist and dietitian, during an inpatient hospitalization, or through a combination of both. The patient can be given the opportunity to wear the pump for several days, using normal saline to master the technical skills associated with pump therapy and to increase the com-

---

Table 7.4. Education for Insulin Pump Use

- Phase 1: Choosing insulin pump therapy (1–2 outpatient visits)
  - Components of insulin pump therapy
  - Advantages and disadvantages of insulin pump therapy
  - Financial requirements
  - Goals of therapy
  - Suitability for insulin pump use, e.g., several-month trial of frequent blood glucose monitoring, trial of multiple daily insulin injections, and/or use of insulin algorithms
- Phase 2: Initiating insulin pump therapy (4–5 days in outpatient clinic or combination of 3–4 outpatient visits and a 3-day hospital stay)
  - Technical components of the insulin pump
  - Blood glucose monitoring technique and accuracy are confirmed
  - Meal planning
  - Symptoms, prevention, and treatment of hypoglycemia
  - Trial of wearing the insulin pump using normal saline (optional)
  - Determination of insulin needs for the prescribed meal plan while using the insulin pump
- Phase 3: Postinitiation of insulin pump therapy (biweekly visits with weekly phone contact for 2–4 mo)
  - Have the patient keep food, blood glucose, and insulin records
  - Focus on mastering blood glucose monitoring, meal planning, and insulin pump operation
  - Fine-tune insulin dosages to achieve blood glucose goals
  - Identify relationships between blood glucose readings and food intake, activity, and insulin
  - Adjust aspects of the regimen to meet lifestyle needs based on patient input
  - Assist patient to integrate the treatment plan into daily life
- Phase 4: Ongoing follow-up (1-h visits every 1–3 mo using all team members)
  - How to interpret blood glucose readings
  - How to adjust insulin for variations in dietary intake and activity
  - How to use the pump to deal with varying situations
  - How to deal with pump-related problems
  - How to adapt treatment recommendations to changes in lifestyle situations
  - How to anticipate situations that could cause alterations in glycemic control
  - How to identify obstacles to implementing treatment recommendations and develop strategies to overcome obstacles
  - How to set and evaluate treatment and blood glucose goals

fort of wearing the pump. The inpatient hospitalization could be a short 3-day stay, during which skills learned as an outpatient are verified and refined and insulin dosages are determined. If pump initiation and education is done on an outpatient basis, several days at the clinic with frequent blood glucose monitoring and close contact with the health-care team will be necessary. The focus during this phase should be on teaching the basic components of insulin pump therapy, including the technical components of the pump, the pump's delivery system for insulin, the meal plan, monitoring of blood glucose, and prevention and treatment of hypoglycemia and hyperglycemia.

The third phase begins after insulin dosages are determined and the patient demonstrates technical competence using the pump. This phase is an intensive period of follow-up lasting 2–6 mo during which the patient masters the skills learned in phase two and integrates those skills into the usual activities of daily life. Visits with some member of the health-care team may take place every 2–3 wk, with weekly phone contact. Blood glucose and food records are kept to assist the patient in learning to plan the meal and to identify relationships between blood glucose levels, insulin dose and timing, dietary intake, and activity. These records also assist the health-care team in modifying insulin doses and the meal plan as needed and determining whether the patient understands all of the components of the treatment plan.

When the insulin dosages are fine-tuned to the patient's meal plan and usual routine and the patient has mastered the components of intensive diabetes management via CSII, phase four of patient education begins. This phase continues throughout the patient's treatment. At each outpatient visit, in addition to non–pump-specific monitoring, the patient's adaptation to pump therapy is evaluated. Education may focus on teaching the patient to

- use the features of the insulin pump to deal with various situations, such as using the temporary basal rate function during exercise, and
- deal with any insulin pump-related problems, including difficulties in keeping the infusion set securely taped in place, infusion site discomfort, and unexplained hyperglycemia.

Table 7.5. Educational Content for Insulin Pump Therapy

- Pump operation
  - Placement of the battery
  - Programming of the meal bolus, basal rate(s), and time
  - Suspension of insulin delivery
  - Programming of temporary basal rate changes
  - Preparation and placement of insulin syringe and infusion set
  - Infusion site care
  - Cleaning and maintenance of the pump
  - Meaning of alarms and how to respond
  - Special programming options
  - Troubleshooting
- Self-monitoring of blood glucose
  - Determine proper technique
  - Confirm accuracy of results
  - Interpret blood glucose readings
  - Set blood glucose goals
- Meal planning and relationship between insulin and food
- Use of insulin algorithms
- Hypoglycemia and hyperglycemia: symptoms, prevention, treatment
- Unexplained hyperglycemia: causes, prevention, identification, treatment
- Sick-day management
- Dealing with exercise
- Options for special occasions
- Insulin regimen when insulin pump use is not desired or pump malfunctions
- Decision making; strategies for dealing with lifestyle situations

IMPLANTABLE INSULIN INFUSION PUMPS

Investigations into the feasibility and safety of implantable insulin-delivery systems began in the 1980s. These investigations resulted in the development of implantable pumps that deliver insulin safely. However, problems with this form of insulin delivery remain, and implantable insulin pumps continue to be experimental and are not commercially available in the United States.

Implantable pumps are disk shaped with a titanium outer casing. They are >9 cm in diameter and weigh 250–300 g. The power source is a lithium chloride battery with a life of 3–5 yr. The reservoir contains 10–15 ml insulin, which is a buffered, surfactant-stabilized human insulin designed to reduce the incidence of insulin aggregation. Insulin is infused in concentrations of U-400 or U-100. An access port to the reservoir allows repeated percutaneous needle punctures for insulin refills. The reservoir must be refilled every 1–3 mo. Microprocessors and electronic devices, including a radio receiver and transmitter, are built into the pump. The implantable insulin pump is programmable to deliver basal rates that can be modified, based on varying daily activities. Boluses are programmed and then delivered by holding an external transmitter over the implanted pump.

The insulin pump is implanted into a subcutaneous pocket in the abdomen under local, spinal, or general anesthesia, depending on patient and physician preference. Insulin is infused through a catheter consisting of an outer layer of silicone rubber and an inner layer of polyethylene. Catheters are placed either intravenously or into the intraperitoneal cavity. For intravenous insulin deliver, the catheter is inserted into the subclavian vein so that the tip of the catheter is located in the superior vena cava.

Evidence to date indicates that implantable insulin pumps function safely. No instances of overdelivery have been reported. The surgical procedure needed for pump implantation is well tolerated, and the incidence of infection is rare. Improvements in glycemic control, with decreases in episodes of severe hypoglycemia, have been reported after pump implantation. In addition, patients indicate satisfaction with this form of insulin delivery.

Problems with implantable insulin pumps still exist, however. Catheter occlusions resulting in a slow down of insulin flow and subsequent hyper-glycemia remain a significant complication. Subclavian vein thrombosis and ventricular arrhythmia have been reported with intravenous catheters. Migration of the catheters has occurred. Early postoperative fluid collections in the pump pocket are common, although these usually resolve spontaneously. The need for surgical procedures requiring anesthesia to correct a problem with a catheter or to replace a pump remains an important concern.

Despite these problems, implantable insulin pumps may represent a step toward better insulin delivery in the future. Combined with a glucose sensor, these devices could be part of a closed-loop system that could safely normalize blood glucose levels and significantly improve the health of patients with diabetes.

BIBLIOGRAPHY

Bending JJ, Pickup JC, Keen H: Frequency of diabetic ketoacidosis and hypoglycemic coma during treatment with continuous subcutaneous insulin infusion: audit of medical care. *Am J Med* 79: 685–91, 1985

Chantelau E, Lange G, Sonnenberg GE, Berger M: Acute cutaneous complications and catheter needle colonization during insulin pump therapy. *Diabetes Care* 10: 478–82, 1987

DCCT Research Group: Epidemiology of severe hypoglycemia in the Diabetes Control and Complications Trial. *Am J Med* 90:450–59, 1991

DCCT Research Group: Implementation of treatment protocols in the Diabetes Control and Complications Trial. *Diabetes Care* 18: 361–76, 1995

Farkas–Hirsch R, Levandoski LA: Implementation of continuous subcutaneous insulin infusion therapy: an overview. *Diabetes Educator* 14:401–406, 1988

Hirsch JI, Wood JH, Thomas RB: Insulin absorption to polyolefin infusion bottles and polyvinyl chloride administration sets. *Am J Hosp Pharm* 38:995–97, 1981

Hirsch RF, Hirsch IB: Continuous subcutaneous insulin infusion: a review of the past and its implementation in the future. *Diabetes Spectrum* 7:80–84, 1994

Lauritzen T, Pramming S, Deckert T, Binder C: Pharmacokinetics of continuous subcutaneous insulin infusion. *Diabetologia* 24:326–29, 1983

Mecklenburg RS, Benson EA, Benson JW Jr, Fredlund PN, Guinn T, Metz RJ, Nielson RL, Sanner CA: Acute complications associated with insulin infusion pump therapy: report of experience with 161 patients. *JAMA* 252:3265–69, 1984

Mecklenburg RS, Guinn TS: Complications of insulin pump therapy: the effect of insulin preparation. *Diabetes Care* 8:367–70, 1985

Peden NR, Braaten JT, McKendry JB: Diabetic ketoacidosis during long-term treatment with continuous subcutaneous insulin infusion. *Diabetes Care* 7:1–5, 1984

Pickup JC, Viberti GC, Bilous RW, Keen H, Alberti KG, Home PD, Binder C: Safety of continuous subcutaneous insulin infusion: metabolic deterioration and glycaemic autoregulation after deliberate cessation of infusion. *Diabetologia* 22:175–79, 1982

Pietri A, Raskin P: Cutaneous complications of chronic continuous subcutaneous insulin infusion therapy. *Diabetes Care* 4:624–27, 1981

Pitt HA, Saudek CD, Zacur HA: Long-term intraperitoneal insulin delivery. *Ann Surg* 216:483–91, 1992

Raskin P: Treatment of insulin-dependent diabetes with portable insulin infusion devices. *Med Clin North Am* 66:1269–83, 1982

Saudek CD, Selam JL, Pitt HA, Waxman K, Rubio M, Jeandidier N, Turner D, Fischell RE, Charles MA: A preliminary trial of the programmable implantable medication system for insulin delivery.

N Engl J Med 321:574–579, 1989

Schade DS, Santiago JV, Skyler JS, Rizza RA: *Intensive Insulin Therapy*. Princeton, NJ, Excerpta Med., 1983

Schiffrin A, Belmonte M: Multiple daily self-glucose monitoring: its essential role in long-term glucose control in insulin-dependent diabetic patients treated with pump and multiple subcutaneous injections. *Diabetes Care* 5:479–84, 1982

Schiffrin A, Parikh S: Accommodating planned exercise in type I diabetic patients on intensive treatment. *Diabetes Care* 8:337–42, 1985

Schiffrin A, Suissa S: Predicting nocturnal hypoglycemia in patients with type I diabetes treated with continuous subcutaneous insulin infusion. *Am J Med* 82:1127–32, 1987

Selam JL, Micossi P, Dunn FL, Nathan DM, Implantable Insulin Pump Trial Study Group: Clinical trial of programmable implantable insulin pump for type I diabetes. *Diabetes Care* 15:877–85, 1992

Simonson DC, Tamborlane WV, Sherwin RS, Smith JD, DeFronzo RA: Improved insulin sensitivity in patients with type I diabetes mellitus after CSII. *Diabetes* 34 (Suppl. 3):80–86, 1985

Skyler JS, Seigler DE, Reeves ML: Optimizing pumped insulin delivery. *Diabetes Care* 5:135–39, 1982

Sonnenberg GE, Kemmer FW, Berger M: Exercise in type I (insulin-dependent) diabetic patients treated with continuous subcutaneous insulin infusion. *Diabetologia* 33:696–703, 1990

Strowig SM: Initiation and management of insulin pump therapy. *Diabetes Educator* 19:50–58, 1993

Teutsch SM, Herman WH, Dwyer DM, Lane JM: Mortality among diabetic patients using continuous subcutaneous insulin infusion pumps. *N Engl J Med* 310:361–68, 1984

Monitoring

Highlights

Monitoring by the Patient
    Blood Glucose
    Urine Ketones
    Record Keeping

Monitoring by the Health-Care Team
    Glycated Hemoglobin
    Hypoglycemia

Monitoring for Long-Term Complications

Highlights
Monitoring

- Regular monitoring is an essential component of any diabetes regimen. During intensive diabetes management, monitoring is even more important and must be done more frequently than during conventional treatment.

- Monitoring during intensive diabetes management must include self-monitoring of blood glucose (SMBG), as well as urine ketone monitoring and careful record keeping (see pageXX and Table 8.1).

- Monitoring of blood glucose during symptoms of hypoglycemia is strongly recommended, as is monitoring before driving an automobile.

- Monitoring of metabolic control by the health-care team should include
    - glycated hemoglobin
    - review of blood glucose
    - summary of hypoglycemia
    - assessment of growth and weight.
These should be done at each visit.

- Glycated hemoglobin results should be discussed with the patient in terms that the patient can understand and with an understanding of the assay used.

- Monitoring for the development and progression of long-term complications of diabetes should be performed at least as proposed by the American Diabetes Association in its Standards of Medical Care for Patients With Diabetes Mellitus (see Table 8.5 and pagesXX).

Monitoring

Regular monitoring is an essential component of any diabetes management regimen. In intensive diabetes management, monitoring is even more important and must be done more frequently than in conventional treatment regimens. This is true for both the medical monitoring performed by the health-care team and the day-to-day monitoring required by the patient. Patient monitoring consists of self-monitoring of blood glucose (SMBG) and urine ketone monitoring. Monitoring by health-care providers includes regular determination of glycated hemoglobin, careful assessment of growth and development (in children) and weight (in adults), careful review of hypoglycemic episodes and related complications, and monitoring for the presence of long-term diabetic complications.

MONITORING BY THE PATIENT

All patients using an intensive diabetes management program must be expected to perform monitoring on a daily basis at home, work, school, or wherever they may be. This monitoring should consist of SMBG, urine ketone testing, and careful record keeping of the results (Table 8.1).

Table 8.1. Patient Monitoring During Intensive Diabetes Management

- Self-monitoring of blood glucose
  - Before each meal
  - At bedtime
  - 0200–0400 at least weekly
  - When symptoms of hypoglycemia occur
  - Before driving
- Urine ketone monitoring
  - During any illness
  - During unexpected or persistent hyperglycemia
  - During times of weight loss (intentional or unexpected)
  - Daily during pregnancy
- Record keeping

Blood Glucose

When implementing an intensive diabetes management regimen, patients often will perform SMBG 4–6 times/day. An inability or unwillingness to perform SMBG should be considered a contraindication for implementing intensive diabetes therapy. The expectation should be for at least 3–4 SMBG determinations each day. An intensive diabetes management regimen rarely can be optimally successful without monitoring blood glucose at least 4 times/day and should not be recommended at all with fewer than 3 blood glucose determinations each day. There are at least 13 systems marketed in the United States for SMBG. Most of these include the use of a meter to determine the glucose result. Factors that should be considered by the health-care provider and the patient when selecting the system most appropriate for their own use are summarized in Table 8.2. *The Buyer's Guide to Diabetes Supplies,* updated yearly and available from the American Diabetes Association, lists available blood glucose meters and testing supplies.

The four essential SMBG determinations for successful implementation of an intensive diabetes management regimen must be made before each meal and before bedtime.

- Premeal measurements are needed to determine the dose of insulin and/or meal or activity alterations required to achieve the target glucose over the next few hours. They also are used to determine patterns of glycemia over time that will guide adjustment of the regimen. It is best that these patterns be observed over periods of at least 3–5 days before making an overall change in the regimen.
- The bedtime blood glucose test is essential in assessing the adequacy of the supper time dose of insulin and is also a key safety component in preventing nocturnal hypoglycemia.
- The morning reading is used to

assess the adequacy of overnight glycemic control.

- In addition, monitoring should include a blood glucose determination at 0200–0400 at least once per week to determine the presence of unrecognized nocturnal hypoglycemia. This is especially true for those in whom the target blood glucose range is near the nondiabetic range or for those in whom nocturnal or severe hypoglycemia or hypoglycemia unawareness has been a problem. Nocturnal monitoring may need to be performed more often than once a week during periods when the basal insulin dose is being adjusted.
- Although postprandial glucose

Table 8.2. Factors to Consider When Selecting Self-Monitoring of Blood Glucose Method

- Accuracy of method from standardized tests
- Range of readings
- Time required to perform test (may vary from 15 s to 2 min)
- Ease of performing test
  - Is washing or wiping the strip required?
  - Is timing by patient required, or is timing automatic?
  - How easy is it to get blood onto strip or device?
- Ease of using meter
  - Is a calibration step required? How often? How easy?
  - Is maintenance and cleaning required? How often? How easy?
- Patient's ability to use the system to achieve accurate results
  - If the patient is color blind, he or she must use a meter
  - Is the patient visually impaired?
  - Is manual dexterity compromised?
- Cost of the strips and the meter
- Manufacturer's warranty: is there a warranty, and how long is it?
- Availability of technical support services and replacement device
- Availability of a memory function on the meter
  - Does the memory also record date and time?
  - How many entries are in the memory?
  - Can the memory be downloaded to a printer or computer system?

---

determinations are not essential on a regular basis, they can be useful in helping to determine the optimal premeal insulin dose and timing needed to keep postprandial blood glucose levels within the target range.

Monitoring blood glucose during symptoms of hypoglycemia is strongly recommended. Because hypoglycemia can occur with few or no early warning symptoms (hypoglycemia unawareness) and autonomic (adrenergic) symptoms can occur in the absence of hypoglycemia, it is best that the presence of hypoglycemia, and the blood glucose level during the occurrence of symptoms, be confirmed by patients. In addition, because some patients' driving ability may be impaired at blood glucose levels higher than those that usually trigger easily recognizable hypoglycemic symptoms, especially in patients with hypoglycemia unawareness and those using intensive diabetes therapy, it is strongly recommended that blood glucose be monitored before driving.

Urine monitoring for glucose is no longer considered useful in the management of type I diabetes and is not recommended as a regular component of self-management. It is inappropriate for those implementing intensive diabetes management.

Urine Ketones

Monitoring for the presence of urinary ketones remains an essential component of diabetes care. Note that there are no commercially available reliable methods for the quick determination of ketones in the blood. There are certain situations in which urine ketone monitoring is necessary for the safe implementation of diabetes therapy, regardless of the type of therapy used (Table 8.1). Whenever the blood glucose level is unexpectedly or repeatedly >240–300 mg/dl (>13.3–16.7 mM), it is recommended that the urine be checked for ketones. The same is true during intercurrent illness, especially a gastrointestinal illness, regardless of the blood glucose result. Illness can trigger diabetic ketoacidosis, which requires rapid identification and intervention to avoid significant illness and possible hospitalization. In addition, ketosis itself can cause abdominal pain and vomiting. For subjects using an insulin pump, ketonuria, especially when present along with hyperglycemia, may indicate failure of the insulin-delivery system. Ketones also should be measured on a regular schedule in patients actively trying to lose weight by calorie restriction. These patients may be on very low doses of insulin to avoid hypoglycemia. If these low doses cause a state of inappropriate underinsulinization, ketosis and ketoacidosis can occur. It is even possible for ketosis to occur without marked hyperglycemia in a patient who is actively dieting to lose weight. Finally, it is recommended that urinary ketones be monitored daily in women who are pregnant.

Record Keeping

Careful and organized recording of the SMBG results should be considered an essential component of intensive diabetes management. Many blood glucose meters have a memory that stores blood glucose values along with the date and time of day and systems to enable downloading of the results to various computerized systems. However, maintenance of a written log is very important. Unless the patients are able to download the results and review them every few days, they would be unable to examine their records in a way that enables them to look for patterns over 3–5 days and then make necessary adjustments in the regimen. It is very useful to record blood glucose values in logs that enable recording of all the results for a given day across a single row, with those for the same time of day over many days lining up in columns. There should be multiple days, or perhaps a week or two, on a single page. This format enables the patient and health-care provider to quickly scan the log. Any given day can be reviewed by looking across a single row of the log. All the results for a given time of day (for example, pre-lunch) can be reviewed by looking down a single column. This is the most effective format for seeing patterns and trends. It is also helpful if the log has spaces for recording insulin doses, hypoglycemic episodes, and additional notes and comments. Some highly conscientious and motivated patients will highlight their blood glucose log with one color for values below the target and with another color for values above the target. Although this approach is not essential, it can be very helpful in observing trends. For example, if at quick glance there are several yellow-highlighted values (when the patient has used yellow to indicate a low blood glucose level), then a lower insulin dose may be needed.

Many blood glucose meters now have the capability to download data into a computerized database for analysis and long-term storage. Use of such computerized databases is not essential to the successful implementation of diabetes care. However, some health-care providers find it helpful to observe SMBG results in one of the various graphic or text formats provided by these computer software systems. Reviewing the results on the computer screen with the patient at the time of a visit can be helpful and educational in some settings.

MONITORING BY THE HEALTH-CARE TEAM

Overall metabolic control in people with diabetes is assessed primarily by four factors:
- the average overall blood glucose level
- the frequency and severity of hypoglycemia
- the adequacy of growth and development in children and weight gain in adults, and
- the plasma lipid levels.

After daily to weekly office visits at the outset of intensive diabetes management when the program is being implemented and adjusted, the patient will require scheduled visits to assess the success (or lack of success) of the program (Table 8.3).

It is common practice to assess a patient's glycemic control and general health status quarterly. This schedule usually is sufficient for the patient using intensive diabetes management after the initial phase of stabilization has passed. At each visit,

- blood glucose monitoring accuracy is checked
- blood glucose data are reviewed
- issues of diet are discussed
- glycated hemoglobin is measured
- body weight is noted
- problems with hypoglycemia are studied, and
- sites of insulin administration are examined.

Glycated Hemoglobin

Glycated hemoglobin testing is an essential component of diabetes management. The level should be measured approximately every 2–3 mo in patients with type I diabetes who are using intensive diabetes management regimens. The results of the glycated hemoglobin test should be provided to patients and discussed with them in terms that can be related to average blood glucose results. Comparison should be made between the glycated hemoglobin value and the recorded SMBG values. Monthly measurements of glycated hemoglobin may be useful during periods of changing diabetes regimens; even though the value may not stabilize for a couple of months, the trend that is apparent after only 1–2 mo is helpful in assessing the adequacy of the regimen.

Glycated hemoglobin can be measured by numerous different methods (Table 8.4.). Knowledge of the method used to determine the glycated hemoglobin level and the normal range for the particular assay used is essential to its appropriate interpretation. Methods available include

- high-performance liquid chromatography (HPLC)
- ion-exchange minicolumns
- affinity chromatography
- immunoassay, and
- colorimetric assays.

In general, HPLC and ion-exchange chromatography separate glycated hemoglobin from normal hemoglobin by their difference in charge. HPLC is specific for HbA_{1c}; the test is precise and reproducible. Ion-exchange minicolumns measure HbA_{1c} as the primary species along with other nongly- cated species, which do not fluctuate with changes in blood glucose and are of no particular significance. However, these other species may fluctuate in other conditions. Ion-exchange minicolumn methods tend to be less precise than HPLC methods. Affinity chromatography methods measure total GHb; this includes HbA_{1c} as well as other glycated species. An immunoassay method that enables the rapid and specific determination of HbA_{1c} using very small quantities of blood has become available.

The translation of glycated hemoglobin into a specific average blood glucose level is imperfect and must be done with a good understanding of the assay method used. Although the normal ranges for HbA_{1c} and GHb may overlap, the values obtained at a given level of glycemia are higher for GHb than for HbA_{1c}. It has been suggested that all glycated hemoglobin assays be standardized and reported in values equiv-

---

Table 8.3. Monitoring Metabolic Control

- Determine glycated hemoglobin at least quarterly in type I diabetes and at least semiannually in type II diabetes
- Review self-monitoring of blood glucose results carefully at every visit, as well as between visits
- Review the frequency, severity, recognition, and treatment of hypoglycemia
- Assess growth and development in children and teenagers and weight in adults
- Take a careful history related to the management of sick days and occurrence of ketoacidosis
- Monitor blood lipids every 5 yr

alent to the HbA$_{1c}$, as measured in the Diabetes Control and Complications Trial. However, such standardization is not yet a reality. Therefore, it is essential that the health-care provider use a single assay method, preferably a single lab, to determine all glycated hemoglobin results in their patients.

Despite these minor drawbacks, the glycated hemoglobin test remains the best indicator of average blood glucose levels over the preceding couple of months. Other measures of protein glycation, particularly fructosamine and glycated albumin, have been suggested as measures of diabetes control over a smaller time span (a few weeks), but these have not come into widespread use and are of limited value in the long-term management of diabetes. They may have a place in short-term follow-up of recently implemented interven-

Table 8.4. Summary of Methods for Determination of Glycated Hemoglobin*

METHOD	ASSAY TYPE	COMPONENT MEASURED	ASSAY INTERFERENCE BY	
			HEMOGLOBIN-OPATHY	NONGLUCOSE ADDUCTS
■ Affinity chromatography (AC)				
Glyc-Affin (Isolab)	AC minicolumn	GHb	No	No
GlycoTest (Pierce)	AC minicolumn	GHb	No	No
Glyco-Tek (Helena)	AC minicolumn	GHb	No	No
Vision GHb (Abbott)	AC column	GHb	No	No
IMx$_{1c}$ (Abbott)	AC	GHb	No	No
CLC330 (Primus)	Affinity HPLC	GHb	No	No
Merck HPLC (Merck)	Affinity HPLC	GHb	No	No
■ Ion-exchange chromatography (IEC)				
Quik-Sep (Isolab)	IEC minicolumn	HbA$_1$	Yes	Yes
HbA$_{1c}$ column (Bio Rad)	IEC minicolumn	HbA$_{1c}$	Yes	Yes
Glyco Hb Quik (Helena)	IEC minicolumn	HbA$_1$	Yes	Yes
Diamat (Bio-Rad)	HPLC	HbA$_{1c}$	Yes	Yes
Variant (Bio-Rad)	HPLC	HbA$_{1c}$	Yes	Yes
Modular (Bio-Rad)	HPLC	HbA$_{1c}$	Yes	Yes
Pharmacia	HPLC	HbA$_{1c}$	Yes	Yes
Menarini	HPLC	HbA$_{1c}$	Yes	Yes
Waters	HPLC	HbA$_{1c}$	Yes	Yes
Biomen	HPLC	HbA$_{1c}$	Yes	Yes
Vydac	HPLC	HbA$_{1c}$	Yes	Yes
■ Immunoassay				
DCA 2000 (Miles)	Immunoassay	HbA$_{1c}$	No	No
Dako test (Novoclone)	Immunoassay	HbA$_{1c}$	Yes	No
Hemoglobin A$_{1c}$ Tina-quant (Boehringer Mannheim)	Immunoassay	HbA$_{1c}$	No	No
■ Electrophoresis				
Glytrak (Corning)	Electrophoresis	HbA$_1$	Yes	Yes
REP Glyco-30 (Helena)	Electrophoresis	HbA$_1$	Yes	Yes
Diatrac HbA$_{1c}$ (Helena)	Electrophoresis	HbA$_{1c}$	Yes	Yes
■ Colorimetric				
Thiobarbituric acid	Colorimetric	GHb	No	No

GHb, total glycated hemoglobin (includes HbA$_{1c}$); HPLC, high-performance liquid chromatography.

* This table may not include all of the available tests. Some tests are in widespread usage; others are used less frequently.

tions to lower blood glucose and as monitoring tools in some short-term intervention studies.

Although the glycated hemoglobin gives reliable information about the average blood glucose level over the preceding 6–12 wk, it still is essential for the health-care provider to review the blood glucose record carefully at each visit and often between visits as well. The use of the telephone or fax is helpful for the between-visit contacts. This review should keep in mind the individualized goals for blood glucose level and should include an overall inspection of the blood glucose values since the last visit, as well as an examination for patterns of hyper- and hypoglycemia. Identification of patterns should trigger a change in regimen. If there is considerable discrepancy between the glycated hemoglobin result and the recorded SMBG values, the reason for this discrepancy should be sought.

Hypoglycemia

Hypoglycemia is a complicating factor of all insulin therapy and is more common during intensive diabetes management. It is essential that the health-care provider review the patient's experience with hypoglycemia at each visit. This review should include an estimate of cause; frequency; symptoms; and recognition, severity, and treatment of hypoglycemia. If hypoglycemia unaware-ness or severe hypoglycemia is occurring, additional education, related to recognition and prevention of hypoglycemia, should be undertaken. If hypoglycemia cannot be avoided, consideration should be given to changing the target blood glucose range, as discussed elsewhere.

MONITORING FOR LONG-TERM COMPLICATIONS

The long-term complications of diabetes mellitus include retinopathy and cataracts; renal insufficiency and hypertension; autonomic and peripheral neuropathy; and macrovascular disease manifested by heart attack, stroke, and peripheral vascular disease. Despite the fact that better glycemic control, using intensive diabetes therapy, delays the onset and slows the progression of retinopathy, nephropathy, and neuropathy and improves the risk factor profile related to macrovascular disease, complications of diabetes have not been eliminated yet. Therefore, monitoring for their presence and appropriate intervention or referral are required (Table 8.5).

Annual comprehensive examination by an eye doctor is recommended for all patients > 12 yr of age with diabetes for > 5 yr; all patients > 30 yr old, regardless of the duration of diabetes; and for any patient with visual symptoms or abnormalities. A fasting lipid profile should be repeated every 5 yr in those whose values fall within acceptable risk levels. It should be repeated yearly in those with abnormal lipid values. Abnormal lipid values should trigger intervention, including dietary counseling, attempts to achieve better glycemic control, and lipid-lowering medication, as indicated. With the socks and shoes removed, the feet should be examined carefully at each visit. The examination should include inspection to assess hygiene and to determine the presence of any ulcers or infection. The assessment also should include a careful history to ascertain the presence of numbness, paresthesia or tingling, or weakness. Pulses should

---

Table 8.5. Monitoring for Long-Term Complications

- Comprehensive dilated eye and visual examination if
  - Age ≥12 yr with duration of diabetes > 5 yr
  - Age > 30 yr, regardless of duration
  - Any visual symptoms/abnormalities
- Monitoring of blood lipids every 5 yr
- Careful examination of the feet (sensation, pulses, reflexes) at each visit
- Careful assessment of blood pressure at each visit
- Annual determination of urinary albumin if duration

be palpated, and reflexes and sensation checked.

Renal status should be monitored regularly. Blood pressure should be taken at each visit. If it is elevated, repeated measures should be taken to confirm the presence of hypertension, and antihypertensive therapy should be implemented. An annual urinalysis should be performed. However, these should not take the place of a urine albumin determination, which should be done yearly in all patients who have had diabetes for >5 yr. Timed collections for albumin are considered the most reliable measure of microalbuminuria. However, if these cannot be obtained, determination of albumin on a randomly obtained spot urine specimen can be helpful as a screening tool. Strips are available that can be used to screen for the presence of elevated urinary albumin. A timed urinary albumin excretion rate should be obtained if the spot urinary albumin screen is elevated. If the timed urinary albumin excretion rate is elevated, it should be repeated. If persistently elevated, intervention should be implemented.

BIBLIOGRAPHY

American Diabetes Association position statement: Standards of medical care for patients with diabetes mellitus. *Diabetes Care* 17: 616–23, 1994

Nutrition Management

Highlights

Goals of Medical Nutrition Therapy

Target Nutrition Recommendations

Strategies for Type I Diabetes

Strategies for Type II Diabetes

Glucose Monitoring and the Nutritional Plan

Hypoglycemia
  Skipping or Delaying Planned Meals or Snacks
  Inappropriate Timing of Insulin Relative to Meals
  Imbalance Between Food and Meal-Related Insulin Dose
  Inadequate Food Supplementation for Exercise
  Consuming Alcohol on an Empty Stomach
  Oral Treatment of Hypoglycemia

Facilitating Nutrition Self-Management
  Meal Planning Approaches for Intensified Management
  Carbohydrate Counting

Weight Gain Associated With Intensive Management

Highlights
Nutrition Management

- Medical nutrition therapy is indispensable to the implementation of all intensified forms of diabetes care.

- The primary goal of medical nutrition therapy is to promote metabolic control, including near-normal blood glucose and lipid control. The plan must provide appropriate food energy (calories), prevent and treat the acute and long-term complications of diabetes, and promote overall healthy via nutritional adequacy.

- Medical nutrition therapy is often the most challenging aspect of diabetes management, leading to recommendations that every person with diabetes consult a registered dietitian knowledgeable in diabetes for a personalized meal plan.

- Target nutrition recommendations
  - are based on development of a personalized plan based on an individual assessment
  - acknowledge evidence that sucrose consumption per se is not destructive of diabetes control, and
  - relegate weight loss in type II diabetes from its previous role as a primary goal of therapy to the status of a strategy for achieving glycemic control.

- In type I diabetes, the meal plan should be based on the patient's usual intake with respect to calories, food selection, and meal timing. The insulin regimen should be fitted to the meal plan and then fine-tuned over time using the results of blood glucose monitoring.

- In type II diabetes, the patient's usual intake should be reviewed and then distributed through the day to avoid large concentrations of calories or carbohydrate. If the patient is overweight, a moderate calorie restriction (250-500 cal) should be instituted in concert with advice regarding physical activity and needed behavioral or lifestyle modifications.

- Blood glucose monitoring is an essential component of all approaches to intensified diabetes management. The joint evaluation of food and glucose records is a powerful tool for control and allows fine-tuning of both the nutrition and medical plans.

- Hypoglycemia is a significant risk of intensified treatment plans. Nutritional factors often play a role in the cause, and therefore the prevention of, hypoglycemia.

- Greater precision of glucose control can be promoted through calibrated treatment of hypo-glycemia, taking into account both the patient's dose response to oral glucose and the current and goal glucose values.

- Meal planning for intensive diabetes management can employ many different nutritional approaches. Carbohydrate counting is particularly well-suited to intensive diabetes management because it allows the most precise matching of insulin with meal-related demand.

- Weight gain may accompany intensive management when excellent glucose control is achieved. This is related to cessation of previous glycosuria, consumption of extra calories to treat hypoglycemia, and the ability to consume a more liberal diet without loss of glucose control. Strategies to prevent gain include reducing calories at the outset of intensive diabetes management when previous control has been poor.

Nutrition Management

Medical nutrition therapy is indispensable in the successful implementation of all forms of diabetes care. Intensive diabetes management adds importance to nutritional aspects of the diabetes-care formula. Those who fully realize the potential of intensification, using physiologic insulin regimens and frequent blood glucose monitoring to consume a diet with greater freedom of choices while maintaining glucose control, can do so only by applying extremely sophisticated nutrition management skills. As demonstrated in the DCCT, extensive individualized training and problem solving are required to support this style of care in patients with insulin-dependent (type I) diabetes.

In considering methods of intensifying the management of people with non-insulin-dependent (type II) diabetes, it is important to note that even minimal nutrition teaching and counseling frequently are missing from the care of these patients. Because insulin use appears to be the major factor that triggers primary care physicians to refer those with type II diabetes for nutritional care, the very diabetes patients for whom nutrition is the primary, if not the only, treatment modality are those least likely to receive any assistance with this component of their management. Clearly, extending appropriate medical nutrition therapy to this often neglected population would represent a major "intensification" of their care.

GOALS OF MEDICAL NUTRITION THERAPY

The overall goal of nutrition therapy in diabetes is to promote metabolic control. Included in this general objective are several specific targets (Table 9.1). Achieving these goals requires dietitians and other professionals to teach and otherwise assist people with diabetes in modifying or managing their nutritional intake relative to many pertinent factors. These elements include medication; exercise; illness and other stresses; and lifestyle considerations such as work or school schedules, family dynamics, personal preferences and motivation, and cultural and religious concerns.

Achieving consistent management or modification of food intake constitutes the most complex and, often, most challenging aspect of diabetes care. The complexity of the task arises from many factors (Table 9.2) and is the reason for current authoritative recommendations that every person with diabetes consult a registered dietitian (RD) knowledgeable about diabetes to obtain an individualized nutrition plan. Because of the inseparable interaction of nutritional intake with medication and exercise in determining blood glucose levels, nutritional care must be fully integrated with other aspects of diabetes management to be effective. This is best accomplished via team care of diabetes, but at the very least requires open communication

---

Table 9.1. Specific Goals of Medical Nutrition Therapy

- Maintain blood glucose levels as near normal as possible by balancing food intake with insulin (either endogenous or exogenous) or oral glucose-lowering medication and activity levels
- Achieve optimal serum lipid levels
- Provide adequate calories for maintaining or attaining reasonable weight for adults and normal growth and development in children, and for meeting increased metabolic needs during pregnancy and recovery from catabolic illness
- Prevent and, as needed, treat the acute and chronic complications of diabetes
- Promote overall health through optimal nutrition, using accepted guidelines for all healthy Americans such as *The Food Guide Pyramid*

Table 9.2. Some Factors That Contribute to the Complexity of Nutritional Care

- The interaction of diabetes nutritional therapy with both normal nutrition and coexisting pathology, such as abnormal lipids, elevated blood pressure, and other health problems
- The need to integrate nutrition into the remainder of the diabetes regimen
- The difficulty inherent in modifying preferred lifelong food behaviors and preferences
- The need for stepwise training to progressively build requisite knowledge and skills
- The dynamic nature of both diabetes and life that demand periodic and creative modification of the food plan to address changing, and often unpredictable, needs and circumstances
- The need for advanced problem-solving skills to permit self-management of such changes
- The need to meet these and other challenges while preserving the patient's autonomy and quality of life

From Brackenridge BP: The role of the dietitian in intensified therapy. *Diabetes Rev* 2:331-37, 1994

---

among the dietitian and other care providers. The depth and quality of nutrition skill needed by patients following intensified regimens can only be developed over a series of encounters dedicated to nutrition teaching and problem solving.

TARGET NUTRITION RECOMMENDATIONS

The American Diabetes Association's target nutrition recommendations for all people with diabetes were revised in 1994 (Table 9.3). These recommendations differ from previous guidelines in several important ways.

- A personalized nutrition prescription should be based on individual assessment and modified, if necessary, on the basis of clinical outcomes. This has replaced specific guidelines for the calorigenic and nutrient composition of one "standard" diet for all people with diabetes. The components, process, and objective of diabetes nutritional assessment are shown in Table 9.4.
- The recommendations acknowledge scientific evidence that sucrose and other simple sugars are not inherently destructive of diabetes control, opening the way for the inclusion of many tradi-

---

Table 9.3. Target Nutrition Recommendations for All People With Diabetes

- Protein to provide 10–20% of calories (~10% for those with nephropathy)
- Saturated fat to provide <10% of calories (<7% for those with elevated LDL)
- Polyunsaturated fat provides ≤10% of calories
- Remaining calories to be divided between carbohydrate and monounsaturated fat, based on medical needs and personal tolerance
- Use of caloric sweeteners, including sucrose, is acceptable. As all carbohydrates, sugars must be accounted for so that the insulin demand that they create is matched to available insulin (whether endogenous or exogenous).
- Fiber (20–35 g/day) and sodium (≤3000 mg/day), levels recommended for the general healthy population
- Cholesterol limited to ≤300 mg/day
- The same precautions regarding alcohol use that apply to the general population also apply to those with diabetes. In addition, alcohol may increase risk for hypoglycemia and therefore should be taken with food by people who use insulin.

From American Diabetes Association position statement: Nutrition recommendations and principles for people with diabetes mellitus. *Diabetes Care* 17:519-22, 1994

tionally "forbidden" foods in diabetes meal plans.

- The guidelines specify a shift in the primary priority for type II diabetes nutritional management from weight loss to glucose, lipid, and blood pressure control.

Implementing the new recommendations requires changing some of the most prevalent methods of delivering diabetes nutrition care. Specifically, standardized diets and simplistic advice to "avoid sugar" and "lose weight," which too often have comprised the totality of nutrition advice, are clearly revealed as inadequate. The guidelines are compatible with a shift to more intensified programs of management for all people with diabetes. A flow chart describing the major steps in the design and implementation of meal plans consistent with the 1994 recommendations is shown in Fig. 9.1.

STRATEGIES FOR TYPE I DIABETES

The following strategies, recommended for all people with type I diabetes, are the starting point for the nutritional component of intensified management in this group. They form the structure of care, regardless of the specific meal planning approach used.

- Base the initial diabetes meal plan on the patient's usual intake with respect to calories, food selection, and meal timing.
- Select an insulin regimen that is compatible with the patient's usual pattern of meals, sleep, and exercise.
- Synchronize insulin with meal times, based on the action time of the preparation(s) used. Monitor blood glucose levels, and adjust the basic insulin doses and regimen as needed for usual intake.
- Monitor glycated hemoglobin, weight, lipids, blood pressure, and other parameters of interest, modifying the initial meal plan as needed to meet goals.

In addition, to optimize blood glu-

Table 9.4. Diabetes Nutritional Assessment

Diabetes nutritional assessment is the process by which information regarding

- biochemical parameters
- anthropometric measures
- physical status
- dietary intake, patterns, and preferences
- medical regimen
- social history, and
- behavior

is gathered and evaluated to

- identify the patient's nutritional and metabolic status and nutrient needs, and
- assess the patient's ability and willingness to follow possible interventions with the goal of developing a personal dietary approach that best meets needs the patient's nutritional, medical, and personal needs.

From Brackenridge BP: The role of the dietitian in intensified therapy. *Diabetes Rev* 2:331-37, 1994

---

cose control and lifestyle flexibility for individuals using intensive insulin regimens, either multiple daily injections (MDI) or continuous subcutaneous insulin infusion (CSII), it is necessary to

- Derive personal algorithms for the interplay of insulin, carbohydrate intake, and exercise so that patients can rationally adjust therapy as needed for deviations from usual patterns.

When a patient initiates intensive diabetes management, the dietitian prescribes a meal plan using a system for quantifying food. The patient should follow the prescribed meal plan until the insulin dosages result in the desired glycemic levels. This usually takes ~1-2 mo. After the optimal insulin dosage for each meal is established, the insulin dose per quantity of food can be determined. As one example, if a patient's meal plan at lunch consists of one Fruit Exchange, one Milk Exchange, three Starch Exchanges, two Meat Exchanges, and two Fat Exchanges (72 g carbohydrate) and the insulin dose for a normal prelunch blood glucose level

Fig. 9.1. Nutritional Management Flow Chart

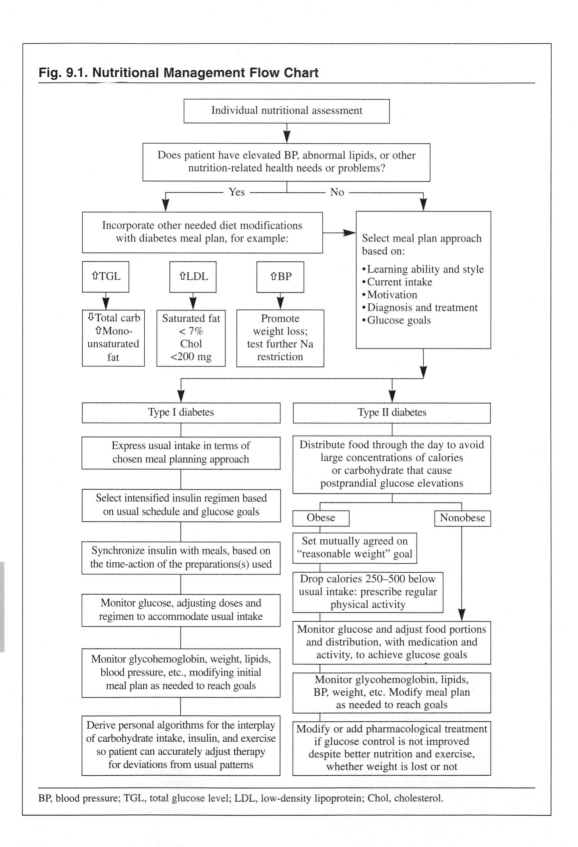

Individual nutritional assessment

Does patient have elevated BP, abnormal lipids, or other nutrition-related health needs or problems?

— Yes ——————— No —

Incorporate other needed diet modifications with diabetes meal plan, for example:

⇧TGL   ⇧LDL   ⇧BP

⇩Total carb ⇧Mono-unsaturated fat | Saturated fat < 7% Chol <200 mg | Promote weight loss; test further Na restriction

Select meal plan approach based on:
- Learning ability and style
- Current intake
- Motivation
- Diagnosis and treatment
- Glucose goals

Type I diabetes

Express usual intake in terms of chosen meal planning approach

Select intensified insulin regimen based on usual schedule and glucose goals

Synchronize insulin with meals, based on the time-action of the preparations(s) used

Monitor glucose, adjusting doses and regimen to accommodate usual intake

Monitor glycohemoglobin, weight, lipids, blood pressure, etc., modifying initial meal plan as needed to reach goals

Derive personal algorithms for the interplay of carbohydrate intake, insulin, and exercise so patient can accurately adjust therapy for deviations from usual patterns

Type II diabetes

Distribute food through the day to avoid large concentrations of calories or carbohydrate that cause postprandial glucose elevations

Obese | Nonobese

Set mutually agreed on "reasonable weight" goal

Drop calories 250–500 below usual intake: prescribe regular physical activity

Monitor glucose and adjust food portions and distribution, with medication and activity, to achieve glucose goals

Monitor glycohemoglobin, lipids, BP, weight, etc. Modify meal plan as needed to reach goals

Modify or add pharmacological treatment if glucose control is not improved despite better nutrition and exercise, whether weight is lost or not

BP, blood pressure; TGL, total glucose level; LDL, low-density lipoprotein; Chol, cholesterol.

is 8 U regular insulin, then the patient requires 1 U insulin for every 9 g carbohydrate, or ~1.5 U for every carbohydrate exchange at lunch. Knowing this, the patient can calculate how much additional insulin to take if a larger meal is consumed. Similarly, less insulin can be taken for a smaller meal. The dosage per quantity of food can be calculated in the same way for breakfast and dinner. If patients need to account for variations in protein intake as well, then three Meat Exchanges can be counted as a Starch Exchange, based on the assumption that 50–60% of the calories from protein contribute to blood glucose levels.

These strategies arise from a strong scientific and behavioral base and describe a much less prescriptive approach than has been common in the past. They acknowledge the difficulty of changing ingrained food habits, the wide range of diet compositions that can be compatible with good diabetes control, and the power that placing the patient's preferences and values at a high priority has to promote adherence to the overall plan of care. Like other aspects of intensified management, they require more provider time and skill to implement than more common approaches, such as first prescribing a standard insulin regimen and then designing the meal regimen to accommodate the insulin schedule and doses.

STRATEGIES FOR TYPE II DIABETES

The primary thrust of medical nutrition therapy in type II diabetes is to achieve glucose, lipid, and blood pressure goals to reduce risk for the chronic complications of diabetes, including cardiovascular disease. In addition to its role in reducing risk for complications, near-normal blood glucose control has been shown to reduce insulin resistance and preserve insulin secretory capacity in type II diabetes. Hypocaloric diets and modest weight loss often improve glycemic control in the short term and, if maintained, can contribute to

long-term improvements. However, because generally effective strategies for long-term maintenance of weight loss are not known, clinicians and patients should direct nutritional strategies primarily toward achieving glucose, lipid, and blood pressure goals. Weight loss has become one of a variety of possible tactics for achieving glucose control, as opposed to being a major goal in itself.

The following strategies form the basis for dietary intervention in all people with type II diabetes. When applied in conjunction with active monitoring of diabetes control as described, they also delineate the nutritional component of intensified management for this group.

- Review the patient's usual intake with respect to total energy, food and carbohydrate distribution throughout the day, fat intake (type and amounts), and food selection.
- Make recommendations regarding improvement in food choices to comprise a nutritionally adequate meal plan with a reduction in total fat and saturated fat, if needed.
- Advise patients regarding cholesterol and sodium intake per guidelines (Table 9.3).
- Distribute food throughout the day to eliminate large concentrations of calories or carbohydrate that may contribute to postprandial glucose elevation.
- If the patient is overweight, negotiate for a moderate calorie restriction <250–500 cal/day below current intake) and regular exercise to help promote modest, gradual weight loss. Calorie restriction is a valuable glucose control strategy for many people with type II diabetes, whether or not weight loss is achieved.
- Monitor blood glucose levels and adjust food distribution, portions, or selection as needed, in concert with medications and exercise, to achieve glucose goals.
- Monitor glycated hemoglobin, lipids, blood pressure, weight, and other parameters of interest, modifying the initial meal plan as needed to meet goals.

Traditionally defined desirable or ideal body weight is no longer used in setting weight goals for diabetes patients. The guideline terminology "reasonable weight" refers to the weight an individual and his or her health-care provider agree can be achieved and maintained, for both the short and the long term.

Modest weight loss, in the magnitude of 5–7 kg regardless of starting weight, is often associated with significant improvement in diabetes control in overweight people with type II diabetes. This outcome is more likely to occur relatively early in the course of the disease, while patients still retain the capacity to produce effective levels of endogenous insulin. In fact, patients who have not experienced an improvement in glucose control with a weight loss in this range are unlikely to see any beneficial effect on glucose control with additional weight loss alone. Persistent fasting hyperglycemia despite a 10-kg weight loss suggests the need for initiation of or changes in pharmacological management of the diabetes. In addition, because glucose control is the primary goal of therapy, an oral glucose-lowering agent or insulin should be considered when glucose control has not improved despite better nutrition and exercise, whether or not weight loss has occurred.

GLUCOSE MONITORING AND THE NUTRITIONAL PLAN

In nutrition, as in other components of diabetes therapy, blood glucose monitoring with appropriate use of the results is the primary factor differentiating conventional from intensive management. Blood glucose monitoring provides the feedback needed to fine-tune the meal plan in concert with exercise, medications, if used, and other relevant factors. When evaluated in relation to food records, blood glucose results can be used to refine the dietary approach in various ways. Postprandial values can guide modification of the

basic meal plan or can be used to tailor the patient's insulin/carbohydrate ratio or insulin-adjustment algorithm. Review of food records in concert with glucose results also reveals the effect of various single foods and food combinations. This is the type of information that is required to increase the patient's flexibility in food choices while preserving glucose control. Some sample monitoring strategies helpful in fine-tuning nutritional care are outlined in Table 9.5.

In patients dependent on endogenous insulin (oral hypoglycemic agents or no pharmacological therapy) and in obese patients using exogenous insulin, the primary strategy to bring postprandial glucose values into the target range is to decrease calories and/or carbohydrate at the problem meal. In people with type I diabetes, the primary strategy for preventing or correcting postprandial glucose elevations is to modify the dose and/or timing of the meal-related insulin dose to match the food consumed. Figure 9.1 schematically illustrates the process of nutrition intervention in intensive management, including the essential role of blood glucose monitoring in evaluating and fine-tuning this aspect of care.

HYPOGLYCEMIA

Nutritional strategies are important to the prevention of hypoglycemia in all people whose diabetes treatment includes a pharmacological agent. Common nutritional factors that contribute to hypoglycemia risk are listed in Table 9.6, and issues and strategies relative to each are discussed below.

Skipping or Delaying Planned Meals or Snacks

Risk of hypoglycemia related to delayed or skipped meals is nonexistent in patients treated by diet only and is very low in insulin pump users whose basal insulin rate(s) is set to maintain stable glucose levels between meals. It is typically lowest for overweight oral agent–treated patients, higher in patients using MDI regimens, and highest in those who use conventional insulin regimens, with a relatively high percentage of their total insulin coming from an intermediate-acting insulin.

These factors should be considered when selecting a pharmacological regi- men. Individuals whose work or other activities makes it difficult to predict or control meal times (e.g., trial lawyers, inpatient staff, or traveling salespersons) will have fewer hypoglycemia problems if placed on regimens that allow more flexibility in meal times.

All patients whose diabetes treatment includes a pharmacological agent should be educated regarding the man-

Table 9.5. Using Blood Glucose Monitoring to Fine-Tune Nutrition Therapy

PATIENT TYPE	PHARMACOLOGIC MANAGEMENT	TIMES OF TESTS	INFORMATION SOUGHT	STRATEGY TO CORRECT ELEVATED VALUE
Type II, obese	None, oral hypoglycemic agent, or insulin	Fasting	Does overnight insulin (endogenous or exogenous) suppress hepatic glucose production and produce desired fasting value?	Reduce total calories; evaluate pharmacological management.
		2-h postprandial or next premeal value	Does available insulin (endogenous or exogenous) cover the meal eaten, producing the desired postprandial value?	Reduce calories and/or carbohydrate in meal plan for preceding meal (if using pattern control) and/or incoming meal. When obesity is present, food reduction and/or increased activity are preferred over medication increases whenever possible.
Type I or type II, nonobese	Insulin	Fasting	Does overnight exogenous insulin suppress heapatic glucose production and produce the desired fasting value?	Adjust dose or timing of insulin acting overnight: review bedtime snack and any other foods eaten overnight.
		2-h postprandial or next premeal value	Is meal-related insulin dose appropriate?	Adjust dose or timing of meal-related insulin; fine-tune patient's insulin adjustment algorithm; evaluate method used to quantify carbohydrate (food values, portions)

Table 9.6. Nutritional Factors Contributing to Hypoglycemia

- Skipping or delaying planned meals or snacks
- Inappropriate timing of insulin relative to meals
- Imbalance between food and meal-related insulin dose due to
  - Inaccurate estimation of food intake when calculating meal-related boluses
  - Consuming less carbohydrate than meal plan without adjusting insulin dose
- Inadequate food supplementation (in absence of medication adjustment) for exercise
- Consuming alcohol without food

agement of meal timing in their particular regimen. Carrying a source of carbohydrate is, of course, a vital self-management behavior for all such patients, and the use of that food to *prevent* hypoglycemia when meal times are unavoidably delayed should be taught.

Inappropriate Timing of Insulin Relative to Meals

The greatest risk for hypoglycemia exists when the peak action of insulin occurs at a time separate from peak glucose release to the bloodstream after a meal. In a common scenario, a patient may take his premeal bolus of regular insulin immediately before eating, resulting in elevated blood glucose values in the immediate postprandial period and a propensity toward hypoglycemia 2–3 h later, when the insulin peaks. Appropriate timing of insulin and meals can be used to reduce this risk.

Introducing an adequate delay, or lag time, between the premeal bolus of conventional human insulin and the meal will produce a better match between insulin action and postprandial glucose availability. A similar benefit is gained from appropriate timing of the lunch meal relative to intermediate-acting insulin injected in the morning. Such timing changes, when needed, can produce better control of

postprandial blood glucose values and reduce risk for between-meal hypoglycemia. Because the action time of specific insulin preparations varies considerably from person to person and is further affected by injection site, exercise, and other factors, blood glucose monitoring should be used to confirm optimal insulin timing relative to meals. Rapid-acting insulin analogs are expected to greatly simplify the timing of meals and insulin for those using premeal boluses by eliminating the need for a delay between the meal-related bolus and the meal. Their rapid clearance from the bloodstream should also reduce risk for between-meal hypoglycemia.

In addition to modifying insulin timing, another strategy for minimizing risk for between-meal hypoglycemia is to include snacks in the meal plan. Regardless of insulin and meal timing, snacks are often needed to prevent hypoglycemia in individuals using conventional split-mixed regimens because of the very broad peak action curves of NPH and lente insulins.

Imbalance Between Food and Meal-Related Insulin Dose

Hypoglycemia will result when the meal-related insulin dose is too large for the actual amount of food eaten. In the intensively managed MDI or CSII patient, who adjusts premeal boluses for anticipated intake, this most often occurs because of errors in estimating food and/or carbohydrate intake when calculating the bolus. Bolus calculations can be based on exchanges, carbohydrate intake, or carbohydrate and protein intake. Whatever method is used, the algorithm employed must be individualized to the patient's response to achieve the best possible glucose control. Most people benefit from a period of weighing and measuring all food eaten to train the eye to accurately estimate portion size. See page 103 for further information on the insulin-carbohydrate ratio.

Some patients can achieve good glucose control without adjusting insulin doses according to the content of individual meals. However, it must be remembered that a static insulin plan requires a static meal plan. If one parameter changes, the other must reflect the change, if control is to be maintained. Even when increasing doses to accommodate extra food intake is not desirable—perhaps because it works against the goal of achieving reasonable weight—guidance should be given for how to prevent hypoglycemia if a smaller-than-normal meal is eaten. Individualized guidelines for insulin reduction could be used, the missing food could be replaced with fruit or fruit juice during the meal in question, or a snack equal to the reduction in the meal could be eaten 2–3 h after the meal.

Inadequate Food Supplementation for Exercise

Blood glucose monitoring is required to calibrate insulin doses and/or carbohydrate intake for exercise to reduce hypoglycemia risk. The decision of whether to adjust food or insulin is determined by the individual's diabetes management goals and is further affected by whether the exercise was planned. When exercise is planned sufficiently in advance, it is preferable to adjust the insulin acting during the period of physical activity to minimize hypoglycemia risk (see MULTIPLE-COMPONENT INSULIN REGIMENS).

If exercise is not planned far enough ahead to modify the relevant insulin dose, a carbohydrate supplement should be taken. Depending on the glucose value at the start of exercise and the intensity and duration of the activity, the supplement may be taken before, during, and/or after exercise. Sample guidelines for carbohydrate supplements for exercise are shown in Table 9.7. These guidelines should be individualized for each patient on the basis of blood glucose monitoring results. When exercise has been intense or prolonged, the risk for hypoglycemia extends into the postexercise period. Therefore, additional snacks may be required in the hours after exercise or before bedtime.

Exercise is central to the overall management of those attempting to reach reasonable body weight. It is obviously preferable to avoid increasing food intake to cover exercise in such individuals. To better support weight management and calorie restriction goals, exercise can be scheduled after meals, because blood glucose values tend to be higher at that time. If this is not possible, or if it is ineffective in preventing hypoglycemia, medication doses should be adjusted downward as needed to allow exercise to proceed without having to unduly increase food intake.

Consuming Alcohol on an Empty Stomach

Alcohol cannot be converted to glu-

Table 9.7. Preexercise Carbohydrate Supplements: Sample Guidelines*

DURATION	INTENSITY		
	MILD	MODERATE	INTENSE
<30 min	None	0–15 g	15–30 g†
30–60 min	10–15 g	15–30 g†	30–60 g†
>60 min	~15 g/h	25–35 g/h†	45–60 g/h or more†

From Walsh J, Roberts R: *Pumping Insulin.* San Diego, CA, Torrey Pines, 1994, p. 90–93
*Based on the average response for 150-lb person. Adjust for individual response based on blood glucose results.
†Anticipatory insulin adjustment is desirable.

cose, inhibits gluconeogenesis, and interferes with the counterregulatory response to insulin-induced hypoglycemia. Through these mechanisms, alcohol taken in the fasting state may contribute to hypoglycemia, especially in people with type I diabetes. Up to two drinks per day *in addition to* usual meals can usually be consumed by those with type I diabetes without adverse effects on blood glucose control. If sweet wines, liqueurs, or drinks made with regular soda pop or fruit juices are consumed, their carbohydrate content may need to be included in calculations for meal-related boluses. However, this should be done with caution because of the extra hypoglycemia risk associated with alcohol use. For this reason, choosing dry wines, light beers, and drinks made with noncaloric mixers may simplify the management of alcohol in people with type I diabetes who choose to drink. Testing blood glucose before going to sleep is a reasonable safety precaution for all people with type I diabetes who have been drinking alcohol.

Alcohol-induced hypoglycemia is less of a risk for people with type II diabetes, largely because of insulin resistance. For people with type II diabetes, who are limiting calorie intake to promote better blood glucose control and/or weight reduction, any alcohol consumed should be substituted for fat in the usual meal plan. Restriction of alcohol may be desired in type II diabetes patients who have dyslipidemia, particularly those with elevated triglycerides.

Oral Treatment of Hypoglycemia

Helping each patient develop a personally calibrated treatment plan for hypoglycemia is a valuable strategy for promoting better blood glucose control. Overtreatment of hypoglycemia is common and is at least partly the result of the patient's not receiving sufficiently specific advice on how to treat their episodes of hypoglycemia. When the same, "Take 15 to 20 grams of carbohydrate," advice is given to all patients, the result will be inadequate treatment in some circumstances and excessive treatment in others. The exact glucose rise produced by a given amount of carbohydrate varies from person to person, primarily a result of differences in body size. Therefore, a given quantity of carbohydrate will generally raise the blood glucose level more in a small person than it will in a larger individual.

Begin with the estimate that each 5 g carbohydrate raises blood glucose ~20 mg/dl (1.1 mM; an approximate value for a 150-lb person). With blood testing, fine-tune this value, based on the patient's response to given amounts of carbohydrate.

- Example: A 100-lb woman having an insulin reaction finds that her blood glucose level is 40 mg/dl. She wants to raise her blood glucose level ~60 mg/dl to 100 mg/dl. She treats the hypoglycemia with 15 g carbohydrate (60 mg/dl desired rise; estimated 20 mg/dl rise for each 5 g carbohydrate = 3; multiply 3 x 5

Table 9.8. Sample Personal Algorithm for Hypoglycemia Treatment

Each 5 grams of carbohydrate raises your blood sugar about *15 mg/dl.*
Your goal blood glucose following treatment of hypoglycemia is about *120 mg/dl.*

If your blood glucose is:	Eat this much carbohydrate:
Less than 40	30 grams
40–50	25 grams
51–60	20 grams
61–80	15 grams
More than 80 with symptoms	5 or 10 grams

g = 15 g). Her blood glucose rises to 145 mg/dl with this treatment. You now know each 5 g carbohydrate raises her blood glucose =35 mg/dl ([105 mg/dl rise/15 mg/dl] x 5 = 35 mg/dl).

Once the personal value is identified, develop an algorithm such as that illustrated in Fig 9.8. The patient can then calibrate treatment of any episode of hypoglycemia based on current blood glucose and target value. Providing an algorithm avoids a potential source of treatment error, because it eliminates the patient's need to perform calculations in a hypoglycemic state.

Virtually any low-fat source of carbohydrate can be used successfully to treat hypoglycemia. Commercially prepared products are higher in available glucose than most high-carbohydrate foods and offer the additional advantage of more precise carbohydrate dosing.

FACILITATING NUTRITION SELF-MANAGEMENT

Achieving the goals of intensive diabetes management requires that outdated concepts of urging people with diabetes to comply with rigid diet prescriptions be abandoned. People with diabetes must be able to make choices and solve problems every day in a changing, and ultimately uncontrollable, environment to keep insulin (endogenous or exogenous), food, and activity in a state of dynamic balance. This requires that each person following an intensified management approach receive the depth and manner of education required to build nutrition self-management skills.

As previously described, this process begins with nutrition assessment to enable the dietitian to tailor medical nutrition therapy to each patient's unique circumstances. The ensuing educational process progresses from the mutual identification of specific goals through appropriate stepwise intervention and is guided throughout by evaluation of the patient's knowledge and skill, as well as by clinical parameters. These processes of assessment and education are similar for every patient, regardless of the specific approach to diabetes meal planning employed.

Meal Planning Approaches for Intensified Management

Several distinct meal planning systems are used in diabetes therapy. Each stresses a different factor, such as calories, portion control, food choices, fat or carbohydrate content, and so on. The DCCT demonstrated that many different approaches to meal planning can be used successfully in intensive management regimens. The four major types of diabetes meal planning systems and the benefits of each are summarized in Table 9.9. The choice of a specific meal planning approach should be based on a review of a variety of factors, including the patient's current intake and food choices, clinical goals, learning style, and desire for flexibility.

The teaching time required for the different approaches varies and should be taken into consideration as well. Effective use of all systems requires that patient teaching and support materials be available. Similarly, all approaches require that a staged program of education be undertaken, progressing from simple concepts of diabetes nutritional management through the more in-depth knowledge that eventually supports nutrition self-management and the informed decision making that it requires.

Carbohydrate Counting

Because dietary carbohydrate is the chief determinant of meal-related insulin demand, accurate identification of the amount of carbohydrate contained in a meal is the key task in finding the appropriate insulin dose for any meal. Carbohydrate counting can be used as the sole meal planning approach, in con-

Table 9.9. Benefits and Drawbacks of Major Types of Meal Planning Systems

SYSTEM TYPE	DESCRIPTION	BENEFITS	DRAWBACKS
General guidelines	Food Guide Pyramid, U.S. dietary guidelines	■ Easy to understand ■ Good initial teaching tools ■ Focus on healthy food choices	■ Low emphasis on portion control complicates coordinating insulin doses with food
Menu planning	Writing out sample menus	■ Specific ■ Simple to use ■ Can guide good choices while patient learns more advanced concepts ■ Can use patient's preferred and available foods	■ Lack of flexibility to respond to unusual circumstances ■ Keeps decision-making in caregiver's hands instead of patient's
Exchange	List that groups foods of similar nutritional content, indicating portions of each that can be substituted to provide variety; accompanied by a meal pattern that indicates the number or range of servings to be eaten from each group each day	■ Include portion control ■ Facilitate calorie adjustment ■ Support materials such as food lists, recipes and menus widely available ■ Multiple nutritional concerns can be incorporated into the meal pattern	■ Exchange concept is difficult for many to understand ■ Time consuming to teach ■ Can be limiting and prescriptive, especially if inadequate education is provided
Counting	Systems that focus on counting amounts of given nutrients: common ones are carbohydrate counting for glucose control and fat counting for calorie control/weight management	■ Allow greatest flexibility in food choices ■ Emphasis is on careful quantifying of food intake ■ Simple to teach and apply because of single topic focus ■ Carbohydrate counting is most precise method for matching insulin to food intake	■ Other nutrition concepts (i.e., healthy food choices or cardiovascular risk reduction) must be taught separately

cert with other systems, to fine-tune blood glucose control. It also can be used by the health-care provider to find the cause of unexplained blood glucose control problems. Because of its particular usefulness in intensive management, carbohydrate counting will be discussed here in greater detail than other approaches.

Initially, carbohydrate counting is implemented as a stable meal plan: a given quantity of carbohydrate to be consumed at each meal and snack. The plan is based on the patient's usual intake. During this initial period, the patient weighs and measures food portions to gain skill in estimating portion sizes and keeps complete food and blood glucose records. This allows identification of his or her insulin-carbohydrate ratio, i.e., the ratio between the grams of carbohydrate eaten and the number of units of insulin required to use them. Once this ratio is known, it can be used to calculate the bolus for any meal or snack of known carbohydrate content. Most individuals with type I diabetes require 1 U of insulin for each 10–15 g carbohydrate. However, such a generalization is not adequate to optimize control. The precise ratio must be found through trial and error by reviewing food records and blood glucose monitoring results.

The amount of carbohydrate in a meal can be estimated in two main ways (Table 9.10). As suggested, some patients find that they achieve better blood glucose control when they also account for the glucose effect of the protein they eat.

Table 9.10. Carbohydrate Counting Methods

METHOD	DESCRIPTION	BOLUS CALCULATION	EASE VS. ACCURACY
Count grams of carbohydrate	Add carbohydrate gram values for all foods eaten to obtain carbohydrate total for meal. Obtain values from reliable food lists, reference books, and food product nutrition labels.	Calculate bolus by dividing the total grams of carbohydrate in the meal by the insulin-carbohydrate ratio.	Very accurate but more time consuming than counting carbohydrates or exchanges. Requires some math skill to add and divide 2- and 3-digit numbers, especially if done mentally.
Count *carbs*	Count servings of starch/bread, fruit, and milk, considering them all to be equal in carbohydrate value. ($\sim$ 15 g/*carb*). Vegetables and meats may or may not be counted (1/3*carb*/ vegetable or meat serving).	Calculate bolus as units/exchange or *carb*.	Easiest method but also the least accurate, because exchanges are based on average values for a whole group of foods. Requires little math skill and uses exchange groups and portions, which patient may know already.

From Brackenridge B, Fredrickson L, Reed C: *Using Carbohydrate Counting to Zero in on Control. Sylmar, CA, MiniMed Tech., 1995*

WEIGHT GAIN ASSOCIATED WITH INTENSIVE MANAGEMENT

Weight gain may accompany intensive management when excellent blood glucose control is achieved. Factors thought to be associated with this phenomenon are failure to compensate for cessation of calories previously lost via glycosuria and consumption of extra calories to treat more frequent episodes of hypoglycemia. If intensively treated individuals, who have achieved excellent glucose control, have a greater array of food choices that can be consumed without loss of glucose control, then they will have the same result from overeating as the rest of the population. They will gain weight. Strategies for preventing weight gain are given in ADVERSE EFFECTS.

BIBLIOGRAPHY

American Association of Diabetes Educators position statement: Individualized meal plans for persons with diabetes. *Diabetes Educator* 1:7, 1981

American Diabetes Association: *Maximizing the Role of Nutrition in Diabetes Management*. Alexandria, VA, Am. Diabetes Assoc., 1994

American Diabetes Association position statement: Nutrition recommendations and principles for people with diabetes mellitus. *Diabetes Care* 17:519–522, 1994

Arnold MS, Stephen CJ, Hess G, Hiss R: Guidelines vs. practice in delivery of diabetes nutrition care. *J Am Diet Assoc* 93:34–39, 1993

Beebe CA: Self blood glucose monitoring: an adjunct to dietary and insulin management of the patient with diabetes. *J Am Diet Assoc* 87:61–65, 1987

Brackenridge B: The role of the dietitian in intensified therapy. *Diabetes Rev* 2:331–37, 1994

Brackenridge BP: Carbohydrate gram counting: a key to accurate mealtime boluses in intensive therapy. *Pract Diabetol* 11:22–28, 1992

DCCT Research Group: Expanded role of the dietitian in the Diabetes Control and Complications Trial: implications for clinical practice. *J Am Diet Assoc* 93:758–67, 1994

DCCT Research Group: Nutrition interventions for intensive therapy in the Diabetes Control and Complications Trial. *J Am Diet Assoc* 93:768–72, 1993

DCCT Research Group: Weight gain associated with intensive therapy in the Diabetes Control and Complications Trial. *Diabetes Care* 11:567–73, 1988

Delahanty LM, Halford BN: The role of diet behaviors in achieving improved glycemic control in intensively treated patients in the Diabetes Control and Complications Trial. *Diabetes Care* 16:1453–58, 1993

Holler HJ, Pastors JG (Eds.): *Meal Planning Approaches for Diabetes Management*. 2nd ed. Chicago, IL, Am Dietetic Assoc., 1994

Lockwood D, Frey ML, Gadish NA, Hiss RG: The biggest problem in diabetes. *Diabetes Educator* 12:30–33, 1986

National Institute of Diabetes and Digestive and Kidney Diseases/National Institutes of Health: *Survey of Physician Practice Behaviors Related to the Treatment of People with Diabetes Mellitus*. Rockville, MD, Prospect Associates, 1990

Walsh J, Roberts R: *Pumping Insulin*. San Diego, CA, Torrey Pines, 1994

Adverse Effects

Highlights

Hypoglycemia
    Prevention

Weight Gain
    Prevention

Infusion Site Infections in Insulin Pump Use

Highlights
Adverse Effects

- Intensive diabetes management has three principal adverse effects
  - hypoglycemia
  - weight gain, and
  - complications of insulin pump use.

- Reducing the risk of hypoglycemia involves reeducating patients concerning warning signs and exercise, increasing frequency of blood glucose monitoring, investigating hypoglycemic episodes for cause, and modifying treatment goals when needed.

- Reducing weight gain involves reducing calorie intake and between-meal snacks, altering strategies for preventing and treatment of hypoglycemia, and increasing the amount of exercise.

- Strategies for reducing insulin infusion site infections are presented in the chapter on INSULIN INFUSION PUMP THERAPY.

Adverse Effects

Every new treatment modality must be evaluated for both potential benefits and potential adverse effects. Intensive management of insulin-dependent (type I) diabetes mellitus has been shown to have both benefits and potential adverse effects. The Diabetes Control and Complications Trial (DCCT) has provided the largest body of data regarding benefits and costs of intensive management, although other sources also have contributed. Intensive therapy has three principal adverse effects: hypoglycemia, weight gain, and complications of insulin pump use (e.g., infusion site infections or increased frequency of diabetic ketoacidosis; see also INSULIN INFUSION PUMP THERAPY).

HYPOGLYCEMIA

In intensive therapy, all forms of hypoglycemia are more frequent, including asymptomatic and mildly symptomatic episodes, severe episodes in which the patient requires the assistance of another person, and the most severe episodes with seizure or loss of consciousness. The increased frequency of hypoglycemia begins immediately with the initiation of intensive management and persists as long as it is continued.

Detailed analyses of the DCCT experience identified factors that predict higher risk of severe hypoglycemia. These included
- male sex
- adolescence
- long duration of diabetes
- high HbA$_{1c}$ before intensification
- low HbA$_{1c}$ during therapy, and
- history of severe hypoglycemia, both before and during intensive management

Although these factors together predict high risk, they are not sufficiently sensitive or specific to be of significant aid in reducing the occurrence of hypoglycemia through patient selection. Nevertheless, risk can be reduced in patients who possess several of these risk factors by modifying the HbA$_{1c}$ goal, the only demonstrated risk factor that can be manipulated. Note that hypoglycemic risk appears to be continuously and inversely related to HbA$_{1c}$, i.e., there is no HbA$_{1c}$ threshold above which risk decreases dramatically.

The syndrome of hypoglycemia unawareness requires special attention. The term describes individuals who lack early warning symptoms of hypoglycemia and whose first symptom may be cognitive impairment. In general, this is a clinical diagnosis based on a careful review of hypoglycemic episodes. Data suggest that glucose thresholds for warning symptoms may be reduced by the occurrence of hypoglycemia. Hypoglycemia unawareness may be partly reversible. That is, awareness may be restored by rigorous avoidance of even mild hypoglycemia or by intensive education to improve the ability to estimate and detect blood glucose level fluctuations.

Prevention

Reducing risk of hypoglycemia during intensive therapy depends on the patient's active self-management. Therefore, intensive therapy should never be offered or advocated without fully informing the patient about the increased risk of hypoglycemia. Although it appears that the risk of hypoglycemia cannot be reduced to zero with available treatment methods, experience suggests that several measures are likely to be helpful (Table 10.1).

Table 10.1. Prevention of Hypoglycemia During Intensive Management

- Reeducate patients about warning symptoms
- Reeducate patients about exercise
- Increase frequency of blood glucose testing; test before driving
- Investigate details of hypoglycemic episodes
- Modify treatment goals for high-risk patients

- Reeducate the patient about the full spectrum of symptoms of hypoglycemia at the initiation of intensive therapy. The nature of the symptoms experienced and the glucose threshold at which symptoms occur often change during intensive management.
- Reeducate the patient about exercise. Patients should learn that routine activities, such as weekend household chores, may represent sufficient extra exercise to precipitate a hypoglycemic event and that vigorous exercise may provoke hypoglycemia as much as 12–24 h after the exercise.
- Increase the frequency of blood glucose testing. Patients should know that frequent blood glucose testing is an essential part of intensive management, both to improve control and to reduce hypoglycemic risk. In addition to the standard four tests per day, additional postprandial tests are often useful, especially during and after a period of increased exercise. For example, a 2-h postprandial blood glucose level of <100 mg/dl (<5.6 mM) indicates a higher than usual risk before the next meal. The importance of blood glucose testing before driving an automobile should always be emphasized.
- Investigate each episode in detail. Identification of the diabetes self-management behaviors that are associated with a given episode will often suggest preventive strategies in similar future circumstances. In addition, through detailed analysis of episodes, patients may recognize

the narrow margin of safety and the minor degree of deviation from routine that may lead to the occurrence of hypoglycemia.

WEIGHT GAIN

The weight gain that accompanies intensive therapy affects patients regardless of age or sex. Most of the weight gain can be accounted for by the reduction of glucosuria and induction of net positive calorie balance associated with improved glycemic control. A small fraction of the weight gain can be attributed to improved metabolic efficiency.

Prevention

Experience suggests that the following strategies may be helpful (Table 10.2).
- Reduce calorie intake at the initiation of intensive management. A detailed nutritional history should be used to develop a meal plan that is 200–400 cal less than that consumed before intensification of therapy.
- Reduce between-meal snacks. For many patients, the traditional between-meal snacks are one of the inconveniences of diabetes management. Elimination of mandatory snacks as a means of reducing calorie intake may be regarded positively by many. A continuing need for snacks between meals may indicate that basal insulin doses are excessive.
- Treat hypoglycemia with glucose. Treating hypoglycemia with foods that contain nonglucose nutrients simply increases calorie intake and often slows the correction of hypoglycemia. Patients should be urged to avoid treating hypoglycemia with such traditional choices as orange juice or cheese and crackers.
- Initiate an exercise program as part of intensive management. The type and amount of exercise should be individualized. Although

Table 10.2. Prevention of Weight Gain During Intensive Management

- Reduce calorie intake by 200–400 kcal/day
- Eliminate between-meal snacks
- Treat hypoglycemia with glucose
- Initiate an exercise program
- Decrease insulin dose for extra exercise
- Teach flexibility in meal planning

the health-care team should aim to keep regimens as simple as possible by avoiding the introduction of demands that are less than essential, some patients are more likely to begin an exercise program that is an integral part of the intensification program.

- Decrease insulin doses for episodes of activity that exceed the daily routines. Traditional dogma has taught patients to eat more when they exercise more than usual, a practice that makes weight control more difficult. With practice and judicious use of blood glucose testing, patients can become skilled at reducing the insulin dose required to offset additional exercise.
- Teach flexibility in meal planning. Patients can be taught to reduce their food intake below their usual meal plan, when this is desirable for convenience or weight control, while making appropriate adjustments in insulin doses. It is often useful to plan occasions when meals and the related meal insulin doses will be reduced or omitted, followed by more frequent blood glucose testing, as an educational exercise.

INFUSION SITE INFECTIONS IN INSULIN PUMP USE

Subcutaneous infections are a clear risk of continuous subcutaneous insulin infusion (CSII). Either cellulitis or frank abscess may be observed. The onset of infection is often heralded by unexpected increase in blood glucose levels, sometimes before any of the classic signs of inflammation occur at the catheter site. Experience suggests that patients who prolong the intervals between changes in catheter and infusion site are more likely to experience infection. Strategies for preventing infections are given in INSULIN INFUSION PUMP THERAPY.

BIBLIOGRAPHY

Cox D, Gonder-Frederick L, Polonsky W, Schlundt D, Julian D, Clarke W: A multicenter evaluation of blood glucose awareness training II. *Diabetes Care* 18:523–28, 1995

Cryer PE: Iatrogenic hypoglycemia as a cause of hypoglycemia-associated autonomic failure in IDDM: a vicious cycle. *Diabetes* 42: 255–60, 1992

Cryer PE, Fisher JN, Shamoon H: Hypoglycemia. *Diabetes Care* 17:734–55, 1994

DCCT Research Group: Epidemiology of severe hypoglycemia in the DCCT. *Am J Med* 90:450–59, 1991

Resources

- American Association of Diabetes Educators
  444 North Michigan Avenue, Suite 1240
  Chicago, IL 60611
  (312) 644-2233/(800) 338-3633
  - AADE administers the test for and maintains a roster of Certifed Diabetes Educators

- American Diabetes Association
  National Service Center
  1660 Duke Street
  Alexandria, VA 22314
  (703) 549-1500/(800) 232-3472
  - **Professional Section Membership**. ADA offers membership for health-care professionals with an interest in diabetes. Members keep abreast of current topics in diabetes through journals, newsletters, scientific meetings, and council membership and receive discounts on ADA books, subscriptions, and meetings.
  - **Recognition**. ADA recognizes diabetes education programs of high quality and maintains a list of programs that have earned Recognition.
  - *Clinical Practice Recommendations*. A collection of the ADA's official position and consensus statements. Published annually as a supplement to *Diabetes Care* and also available for single or bulk purchase.
  - *The Buyer's Guide to Diabetes Products*. Published annually in *Diabetes Forecast*, ADA's monthly magazine for general members. Available for single or bulk purchase.
  - **American Diabetes Association Books**. ADA publishes many books for health-care professionals as well as for diabetes patients. A free catalog listing all books for sale is available through the ADA National Service Center. Some books that may be of interest to health-care professionals are
    - *Maximizing the Role of Nutrition in Diabetes Management*
    - *Medical Management of Insulin-Dependent (Type I) Diabetes*
    - *Medical Management of Non-Insulin-Dependent (Type II) Diabetes*
    - *Medical Management of Pregnancy Complicated by Diabetes*, and
    - *Diabetes Education Goals*.
  - Some books that may be helpful for intensively managed patients are
    - *101 Tips for Improving Your Blood Sugar*
    - *Managing Diabetes on a Budget*
    - *The Take-Charge Guide to Type I Diabetes*, and
    - *The Fitness Book: For People With Diabetes*.

Index

A

Adherence, helping patients with, 37–38
Alcoholic beverages, 99–100
American Diabetes Association (ADA), 13, 36, 192
  Clinical Practice Recommendations, 15
  nutrition management goals, 92–93
  Recognition program, 18
Assessment of treatment, 13, 12
  office methods, 83–87
  glycated hemoglobin, 84–86
  self-monitoring, 81–84
    blood glucose, 81–82
    record-keeping, 83
    urine ketones, 82–83

B

Basal insulin, 1, 67-69
Behavioral issues, 14, 31–39, 43–44
Behavior change, supporting, 38–39
ß-Blockers, 45
Biguanides, 6
Blood glucose levels. *See also* Glucose; Self-monitoring of blood glucose levels (SMBG)
  monitoring, 81–82, 93
  testing frequency, 69, 81
  using results to vary insulin dosage, 62, 63, 69
Bolus insulin, 1, 67-70, 98
Brittle diabetes, 1, 46

C

Catecholamines, 9
Carbohydrate, 7, 68, 93, 95, 99, 103

Carbohydrate counting,
  intensive management in, 101, 103
Children, glycemic goal modification in, 48
Cholesterol, dietary, 94, 95
Closed-loop insulin delivery, 1
Communication, 13
Complications,
  helping patients cope with, 36–37
  impact on intensive management, 5, 6, 45
  monitoring for, 86–87
Continuous subcutaneous insulin infusion (CSII), 58, 67–77, 93, 98
  basal infusion programming, 67–70
  benefits of, 67
  method of insulin delivery, 67
  safety features, 67
Cortisol, 9
Counterregulation,
  hormones in, 8, 100
  response, 34

D

Dawn phenomenon, 57, 59, 66, 67–68
Depression, 33
Diabetes Control and Complications Trial (DCCT), 5, 31, 36, 85, 91, 101, 107
Diabetic ketoacidosis (DKA), 5, 46, 71-72, 107
Diet. *See* Nutrition
Dyslipidemia, 100

E

Eating,
  disorders, 33
  patterns, 34, 93

Education, self-management, 21-27, 74
  assessment, 22
  commitment, 26
  continuing, 21
  curriculum, 22, 23, 24
  evaluating and documenting, 25-6, 27
  environment, 22–23
  goals, 23
  insulin infusion pump, 74–76
  motivation, 25
  negotiation, 25
  nutrition, 101
  sequencing of classes, 23
  pump, 74–76
  setting, 22–23
  strategies, 25
  teacher qualities, 23
Exercise,
  calorie intake adjustment, 99
  hypoglycemia, 99, 108
  insulin adjustment for, 62, 68, 70
  insulin pump use and, 73–74
  personal algorithms and, 93
  SMBG and, 62
  type II diabetes, in, 6
Euglycemic control, 1
Eye disease, 5

F

Family, 14, 73
Fat,
  metabolism, 7–8
  nutrition, 92, 95
Fuel metabolism, 7–9
  regulation of, 8–9

G

Glucagon, 9, 24
Glucogenolysis, 8
Gluconeogenesis, 8, 100

Glucose metabolism, 7–8
Glucose treatment, 108
Glycated hemoglobin concentration,
  goals, 26, 47
  level, as risk factor for hypoglycemia, 107
  measurement of, 84
  methods to determine, 84–85
Glycemic,
  control, 1, 33, 44, 68
  goals,
    benefits and risks, 48
    modifying, 47–48
Growth hormone, 9

H

Health belief model, 43
Health-care team. *See* Team, multidisciplinary
Hemoglobin, glycated. *See* Glycated hemoglobin concentration
Hormone regulation, 8–9
Hyperglycemia,
  correction of, 70–71
  fasting, 96
  unexplained, 71–73
Hypoglycemia, 96–101
  alcohol-induced, 100
  carbohydrate to treat, 101
  exercise-induced, 108
  increased risk of, 5, 86, 107
  insulin regimen, 98
  nutrition, and, 96–100
  patient education, 22, 24
  preventing, 107–108
  pump therapy, in, 73
  risk reduction, 73, 107
  SMBG, 108
  treatment, patient guidelines, 100–101
  unawareness, 1, 5, 37, 86, 107

I

Implantable peritoneal delivery system, 1, 76–77
Infection, in insulin pump therapy, 71, 109
Insulin,
  absorption, 55
  action,
    onset, 53
    peak, 53
  adjusting doses, 68, 95, 97–98, 109
  analog, fast-acting, 56
  calculating doses, 60, 68–70
  carbohydrate ratio, 103
  continuous subcutaneous insulin infusion, 67–77
  function, 8
  injection,
    devices, 56, 64
    sites, 55
  injectors, 64
  intensive regimens,
    algorithm usage, 60–61, 69
  intermediate-acting, 53–55, 57, 98
  lente, 53–54
  long-acting, 54
  mixtures, 54
  normal glucose homeostasis, 8
  NPH (isophane), 53–54
  preparations, 53–54
    duration of action, 53
    mixing insulins, 54
  pen, 64
  pharmacology, 53
  pumps, 67–77
    implantable, 76–77
  rapid onset, 53–54
  regimens,
    less flexible, 58–69
    multi-component, 56–59
    specific flexible, 57–58
  resistance, 95
  regular, 53, 68
    stability and miscibility, 54
  supplements, 61
  ultralente, 57
Insulin-dependent (type I) diabetes mellitus, 1
  intensive management for, 5–7, 44–45
  nutrition management, 93–95
Insulin infusion pump therapy,
  basal rate evaluation during, 69
  blood glucose monitoring during, 69, 70
  contingencies to pump use, 73
  correction, 73
  dosage calculations, 68
  hyperglycemia correction,
    supplemental insulin, 70, 71
  hypoglycemia, 73
    avoidance, 73
    blood glucose monitoring, 73
    insulin adjustments,
    diet variations, for, 70
    exercise, during, 70
    illness, during, 70
  insulin algorithms, 69
  insulin schedule, 68
  patient education, 74–76
    educational content, 76
    phases of, 75
  patient selection criteria,
    financial resources, 74
    intellectual ability, 74
    medical indications, 74
    physical ability, 74
  reasons for, 68
  removal, periodic, 74
  risks,
    hyperglycemia, unexplained, 71–73
    skin infection, 71
      avoidance, 71
  urine ketone monitoring during, 70, 73

wearing the pump,
  exercise, during, 73
  sexual activity, during, 74
Insulin infusion sets, 71
Insulin therapy,
  basal, 57
  flexible regimen, 57
  dosage requirements, 68
  initial dose, 60
  prandial, 56
Intensive therapy, 1
  adverse effects, 107–109
  benefits, 5
  candidates for, 22
  collaboration, 17
  communication, 17
  compliance, 31
  components, 5
  contraindications, 6
  education curriculum, 24
  goals, 46–48
  indications, 6
  meetings, 17
  metabolic considerations, 9
  patient,
    characteristics, 45
    commitment, 33
    stability, 31
  patients with type I diabetes, 44
  patients with type II diabetes, 45
  pattern-adjustment action plan, 63
  physiological basis of, 7
  pregnancy during, 6
  preprandial action plan, 62
  risks, 5, 15, 107–109
  split-and-mixed program, 59
  team, 13–18
  treatment strategy problems, 45

K

Ketoacidosis. *See* Diabetic
ketoacidosis (DKA)
Ketones. *See* Urine tests; *See also* Assessment of treatment

L

Lag time, 1, 98
Lipids. *See also* Fat
  abnormalities, 100
Lipoprotein metabolism, 5

M

Meal planning, 93, 101–102
Meals. *See* Nutrition management
Metabolic control, 91
Monitoring, 81–87
  glucose, 95, 96
    bedtime, 81
    morning, 81–82
    overnight, 82
    postprandial, 82
    premeal, 81
  glycated hemoglobin, 84, 93, 95
  health-care team–performed, 83
  lipids, 86, 93, 95
  long-term complications, for, 86
  metabolic control, 86
  office methods, 83–87
    glycated hemoglobin, 84
  patient-performed,
    recording results, 83
    SMBG, 81–82
    urine glucose testing, 82
    urine ketones testing, 82
  renal status, 87
Multiple daily insulin injec tions (MDI), 1, 6, 68, 93
Multiple-component insulin regimens, 56, 97–98

N

Nephropathy, 5
Non-insulin-dependent (type II) diabetes mellitus, 1
  intensive management for, 6–7, 45–46, 48
  nutrition management, 95–96
  weight reduction, 95
Nutrition management, 6, 91–104
  adjustments, 97
  assessment, 93
  calories, 108
  carbohydrates, 7, 68, 93, 95, 105
  glucose monitoring, 96
  goals, 91
  meal planning, 93, 109
  nonglucose nutrients, 108
  patients with type I diabetes, in, 93
  patients with type II diabetes, in, 91, 95
  personal nutrition prescription, 92
  protein, 98
  recommendations, 92
  snacks, 96, 98–99, 108
  sodium, 95
  sucrose, 92
  therapy, 95
  weight reduction, 95

O

Open-loop insulin delivery, 1
Oral hypoglycemic agents, 96, 100

P

Patient,
  abilities, 43–4
  adherence, 37
  behavior change support, 38

  commitment, 14, 44
  communication with team, 17
  compliance screening, 31
  motivation, 32, 43
  practicing behavior, 31–32, 34
  psychological,
    assessment, 32–33
    illness, 32
  readiness, 14, 21
  resources, 44
  responsibilities, 15
  selection criteria, 43–9
    for pump, 74
  self-care, 13–14
  skills, 13
Physical activity. *See* Exercise
Pregnancy,
  glycemic goal modification, 47
  intensive management for, 6
Protein. *See also* Nutrition
  metabolism, 7
Psychosocial adjustments,
  adherence, long-term, 37–38
  barriers to self-care, 38
  behavior change, supporting, 38–39
  coping, 35, 36–37
  families, 32, 34, 36
  referral to mental health professionals, 35–36, 38
  referral to specialists, 35–36
  stress, 33–35
Psychosocial support resources, 35

R

Responsibilities, for diabetes management,
  patient, 14–15
  health-care providers, 15–16
Retinopathy, 5

S

Self-management, 21–27
Self-monitoring of blood glucose (SMBG), 81
  frequency of, 81
  record-keeping, 83
Stress,
  assessing, 33
  effects of chronic, 34
  intervention strategies, 34
  psychosocial adjustments, 33–35
Sucrose, 92–93
Sulfonylurea drugs. *See* Oral hypoglycemic agents
Support, for patients, 35, 43, 44

T

Team, multidisciplinary, 1, 3
  characteristics, 16
  communication, 13, 37
  composition, 16
  effectiveness, 17
  function, 13
  management, 13
  responsibilities, 15, 16
  roles, 16, 18
Treatment plan, 14

U

Urine glucose determinations, 82
Urine ketone monitoring, 82

W

Weight gain, 5, 104, 107–108
Weight reduction, **95–96**
  diet, 95
  hyperglycemia despite, 96
  physical activity and, 99